VALUE-BASED HEALTH CARE

Linking Finance and Quality

YOSEF D. DLUGACZ

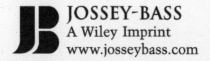

JOSSEY-BASS
A Wiley Imprint
www.josseybass.com

Jossey-Bass books and products are available through most bookstores. To contact Jossey-Bass directly call our Customer Care Department within the U.S. at 800-956-7739, outside the U.S. at 317-572-3986, or fax 317-572-4002.

Jossey-Bass also publishes its books in a variety of electronic formats. Some content that appears in print may not be available in electronic books.

Library of Congress Cataloging-in-Publication Data

Dlugacz, Yosef D., 1947-
    Value-based health care : linking finance and quality / Yosef D. Dlugacz. — 1st ed.
        p.   cm.
    Includes bibliographical references and index.
    ISBN 978-0-470-28167-3 (pbk.)
    1. Medical care—United States—Quality control. 2. Medical economics. I. Title.
    RA399.A3D58 2010
    362.1068'1—dc22

                                                            2009021529

Printed in the United States of America
FIRST EDITION

PB Printing   10 9 8 7 6 5 4

CONTENTS

PART TWO
GETTING DOWN TO BUSINESS

FIGURES AND TABLES

FIGURES

TABLES

PREFACE

As I travel around the country and internationally, speaking to health care professionals, policymakers, and administrative leaders about quality management, I have come to realize how many are unfamiliar with the new concepts of value and value-based purchasing and the relationship between these concepts and quality care, organizational efficiency, and financial success. I am writing this book in order to explain these relationships, especially for those individuals who will be in a position to influence the future of the delivery of care in health care organizations.

In the past when I advocated for performance improvement processes, support came primarily from clinicians and the regulatory agencies. Today, as new processes for improvement are being designed, the C suite has become interested and involved. CEOs and CFOs are beginning to realize that concepts of waste and redundancy in care involve correlations between costs and expenses on the one hand and poor processes and outcomes on the other. Happily, I am beginning to be asked how quality management can help to transform organizations to meet the challenge of value and value-based purchasing. Those who spend money on health care, whether individual patients or large organizations who purchase coverage for thousands of people, are insisting that they get value for their expenditures. Value means good outcomes. Good outcomes require quality management tools, techniques, and processes. Leaders realize that their organizations will fail if they do not provide their patients with value.

Attaching a financial benefit to compliance with quality indicators, as the Centers for Medicare and Medicaid Services and other national organizations are doing, will reinforce the importance of introducing quality oversight into the processes of care. Many administrators still regard compliance with quality indicators as an unnecessary expense and an annoying waste of time. As concepts of value evolve, these same administrators are learning how quality management can increase efficiency and reduce unnecessary expense. By improving care and minimizing errors, organizations receive positive media attention and increased market share. By learning to think about health care as a business, leaders are beginning to take quality management more seriously.

As the senior vice president and chief of clinical quality, education and research for the Krasnoff Quality Management Institute of the North Shore-LIJ Health System, I am in a position to design and implement processes that improve patient safety and reduce unnecessary expenses. Clients of the institute—hospitals and health care systems—ask us to help them develop a strong quality management infrastructure that will improve processes and reduce unnecessary expenses. They are impressed with improved processes that result in fewer excess days for length of stay, better turnaround time in the operating rooms, improved throughput from the emergency department through discharge, and more streamlined purchasing. That is, they see the advantage of planning, data collection, performance improvement, communication, and education about quality management. As organizational inefficiencies improve and the delivery of care results in improved outcomes, administrators and financial professionals realize the benefit to the organization. I hope this volume will illuminate the link between quality and finance for everyone invested in improving health care delivery, patients and professionals alike.

Great Neck, New York   Yosef D. Dlugacz
January 2009

ACKNOWLEDGMENTS

This book is a product of my many years in health care and my association with professionals who have generously shared with me their devotion to quality patient care and their belief that sustained improvements are possible.

I want to thank, in particular, Michael Dowling, president and CEO of the North Shore-LIJ Health System (NS-LIJHS); Mark Solazzo, senior vice president and chief operating officer (NS-LIJHS); Gene Tangney, senior vice president and chief administrative officer (NS-LIJHS); and Mark Claster, Trustee (NS-LIJHS) for their support of the Krasnoff Quality Management Institute and their belief in the value of quality management.

The Krasnoff Institute owes its success to the many professionals who work tirelessly to improve the quality of care in the organizations with which we work. To Carolyn Sweetapple, Cathy Besthoff, Anne Marie Fried, Charles Cal, Jackie Kostic, and Mary Chaber, nurses whose expertise in business management, quality processes, regulatory requirements, utilization, nursing excellence, and education have proved invaluable, many thanks. Marcella De Geronimo and her outstanding staff of data analysts, Roshan Hussain, Nimmy Mathew, Peter Deng, Liz Ciampa, Christina Cheung, Carol Cross, and Ann Eichorn, have provided me with sophisticated information and reports that have enabled me to convince reluctant physicians and administrators about the value of quality data. Thanks also to Robert Silverman, MD, for his commitment to quality research and to his work with the Institute. My son, Hillel Dlugacz, contributed his time and his artistic talent to the cover. Working together is a pleasure and makes me proud.

Special thanks to Debi Baker, for her administrative ability and her graphic design talent, and to Quiana Binns for her clerical support. Joyce Guerriere has made it her business to assist me administratively with diligence and personalized attention. I could not manage without her.

I wish to express my gratitude to the publishing staff at Jossey-Bass, especially Andy Pasternack, who have been supportive of my efforts and generous with their professional advice throughout the years. Working with them has been a pleasure.

To Alice Greenwood, my friend and colleague, who has become my personal trainer of the mind, encouraging me to stretch myself intellectually and who challenges me to be my most productive, coherent and articulate self, I want to express my gratitude and my love.

My wonderful family, Doris, Adam, Stacey, Kylie, Stefanie, and Hillel, has put up with my travels, my long hours, and my many working weekends with understanding, support, and love. Every day I feel how lucky I am to have been so blessed.

THE AUTHOR

Yosef D. Dlugacz, PhD, is the senior vice president and chief of clinical quality, education, and research of the Krasnoff Quality Management Institute of the North Shore-LIJ Health System. The goal of the Institute is to bridge the gap between theoretical knowledge learned in the academic setting and the realities of applying quality management methods in today's health care environment. With decades of experience dealing with process variables and educating professionals and the community about the importance of integrating quality methods into the delivery of care to improve health outcomes, Dlugacz's research focuses on developing models that link quality, safety, good clinical outcomes, and financial success for increased value and improved efficiencies. Dlugacz collaborates with other professionals and organizations to be at the forefront of the national agenda in improving health care services.

Dlugacz's methodologies have been praised nationally and internationally. His academic appointments include Adjunct Associate Professor of Medicine of the New York Medical College; Adjunct Research Professor at New York University; Visiting Professor to Beijing University's MBA Program; Executive in Residence, Hofstra University Frank G. Zarb School of Business; and Adjunct Professor of Management at Baruch/Mount Sinai MBA Program in Health Care Administration, City University of New York. He has appeared in numerous national audio and video teleconferences promoting quality and safety.

Dlugacz has published widely in health care and quality management journals on a variety of clinical care and quality topics. Recently, the Healthcare Financial Management Association published his article "High-Quality Care Reaps Financial Rewards" in their Strategic Financial Planning publication. His book, *The Quality Handbook for Health Care Organizations: A Manager's Guide to Tools and Programs* (Jossey-Bass, 2004), has been praised as a valuable text for new quality professionals. His book, *Measuring Health Care: Using Quality Data for Operational, Practical, and Clinical Improvement* (Jossey-Bass, 2006), helps to educate professionals about the relationship between quality care and financial success. He was invited to write the foreword for the Joint Commission Resources publication, *Getting the Board on Board: What Your Board Needs to Know About Quality and Patient Safety (2007).*

For Kylie Madeleine Dlugacz, my first grandchild,
who enriches my life every day

INTRODUCTION

Unless you have just recently landed on this planet, you are aware that health care in the United States is undergoing dramatic changes. And you probably also realize that health care organizations are failing—clinically, organizationally, and financially—which is precisely why things have to change.

Shockingly, patient care has been defined as "unsafe," with infections, for example, running rampant through hospitals, causing serious harm to patients, and costing organizations a great deal of money and time to rally the resources necessary to address these hospital-acquired infections. Errors—that is, avoidable mistakes, such as giving the wrong dosage of medicine or operating on the wrong part of a patient's body—are now being commonly recognized, again resulting in great harm and expense. As health care organizations have expanded and grown and also have become monsters of their own making, their financial situation has grown correspondingly grim. Furthermore, the population is sicker than ever before, with chronic diseases such as diabetes and heart disease on the increase, requiring constant and expensive interventions. The patient population is also aging, which means that patients come into hospitals with multiple problems and conditions and in somewhat vulnerable physical health. Today's health care environment must address all of these issues. Everyone—health care leaders, governmental agencies, and private insurers—is looking to make a change to repair the clinical, financial, and public relations damage.

Money is driving the change. The carrot of reimbursement and the stick of nonpayment will cause a cultural change that will define value to the patient as not being hurt (that is, being safe) while he or she is in a hospital. Health care organizations still receive reimbursement on the basis of providing treatment. If a hospital patient needs a reoperation or acquires an infection or falls and needs treatment for the resulting injury, the hospital is paid for those services rendered. If a patient is allowed to remain immobile and develops a decubitus ulcer (also known as a pressure injury or bed sore) and that ulcer becomes infected and the patient is medicated for sepsis and requires ICU care, the hospital gets paid. In other words, no matter whether the care is good or bad, the hospital gets paid. Payment is based on volume, the diagnosis, and the procedures required (called the case mix) and also on the length of stay (LOS), the number of days the patient remains in the hospital.

In the past few years, however, the Centers for Medicare and Medicaid Services (CMS), the agency that reimburses hospitals for health care, and other governmental agencies have realized that in effect they were rewarding poor care and the complications of poor care. Now CMS has determined to change things, to reward value and to penalize poor care. For example, methods such as turning the patient to reduce the rate of decubitus ulcers and well-defined processes to help to eliminate these wounds do exist. Yet in today's health care environment, they are still a problem. However, now that CMS has attached a value to reducing this problem, organizations will take more steps to improve processes. Simply put, organizations that provide good care will survive; others will not.

The government has stepped in to encourage hospitals to adopt safer practices through offering financial incentives to hospitals that can document that they have met specific and defined quality measures, such as giving aspirin to heart attack victims or reducing the rate of decubitus ulcers. In the near future, if this trend continues, all reimbursements will be based on performance measures. Medicare calls this pay-for-performance initiative *value-based purchasing*. The idea is to give doctors and hospitals incentives to improve and to give patients value for their health care dollar. The media have also joined the effort and are publishing "report cards" on hospital care so that consumers can be aware and can make intelligent choices for themselves, and the Medicare web site supplies potential health care consumers with comparative data showing how specific hospitals rank on important quality measures.

The government is representing the public in demanding value for health care services. Therefore, hospitals, if they are to survive, have to provide value as their product to their consumers (the patients). It is no longer enough to hire physicians with good credentials and to purchase expensive equipment and then call yourself a "good" hospital. Value, defined as the efficient and effective delivery of good services, must be woven into the entire fabric of the organization, into every process and procedure, department, and service. This book addresses the issue of value in health care: how it can be defined, measured, assessed, and incorporated into the organizational process of the delivery of safe patient care. It also talks about the role and responsibilities of the governing board and the organizational leaders, both clinical and administrative, in determining value for health care spending, and provides information about the relationship between quality and finance. Clearly, improvements in quality lead to improvements in cost management, but many leaders in the health care field, even if they have good intentions, have no idea how to operationalize these improvements. This book should help them realize their goals.

By using quality management methodologies, hospital and health care leaders can link safe care to financial success. Obviously, if you do not make mistakes, you do not have to spend money to correct them. Under the new standards, if a patient requires a reoperation because the initial operation was not performed properly, no one gets paid. Moreover, the expensive resource of the operating room must be used for the reoperation, preventing a paying patient from using the service. If infections and their complications are reduced, the expensive resource of the ICU is avoided. If processes are in place to control unintended consequences, such as falls, then follow-up expenses are also controlled.

When patients are managed properly and care is delivered intelligently, with consistent attention to a method of monitoring care, then everyone benefits and the service delivered is valuable to the patient and productive to the organization. When care is efficient, LOS for patients is shorter than it is when patients acquire unnecessary complications from their hospital stay. When certain conditions can be managed on an outpatient basis, there is less expense for patient, hospital, and insurer. Good care leads to good finances. The concepts presented in this book will help the reader understand the relationship between method and outcome, how quality methods help to produce good outcomes, and how good outcomes lead to value. Quality methods connect operations and the budget and can predict patient outcomes.

Traditionally, there has been a separation between administrative duties and clinical practice, with the physicians in complete control of the delivery of care. Operations, quality management, and budget were considered independent entities, with no connecting corridors, so to speak. That approach is entirely unworkable in today's health care environment. If the CEO does not see that good quality leads to good outcomes that in turn lead to a good bottom line, the organization will fail. If administrative leaders do not have a method for monitoring and improving services and also an approach that develops an effective communication process between administrative and clinical staff, the organization will suffer financially.

Rarely are finance and operations appropriately linked. For example, a member of the board or the CEO might ask why the budget goals have not been met. The financial officer might point to operations to answer the question, saying that LOS is too long or that staffing salaries are too high. However, the question that the board or CEO should ask is, what processes can be used to increase the quality of care so that expenses can be successfully predicted? More specifically, what algorithms for care are in practice? What discharge plans are efficient? Are patients accurately assessed to determine whether they need end-of-life care rather than ICU care? Is the level of competency among the staff appropriate?

Today, these questions must be asked. Today, registered nurses and physicians are enrolling in MBA programs. Today, the silo approach to education is a disservice to everyone involved in health care. Today, the entire scope of care must be considered as a whole. With time, these new educational programs will transform the hospital culture from a focus on caring (treatment) to a focus on curing (outcomes).

The idea of establishing a method to continuously monitor the delivery of care for specific patient populations and particular services is foreign to many leaders. Without such a method, and one that is accepted and internalized by everyone involved in the hospital, the financial picture will remain grim. Quality variables provide such a method, and connect operations, the budget, and patient outcomes. Experts in organizational processes underline the importance of a leadership commitment to making change in order for change to be made. This is as true for health care organizations as it is for automobile manufacturers. Involvement has to move past the boardroom and past the budget to the bedside. Only then can the "product" of the industry increase in value.

For those professionals working in health care and for students who hope to make an impact on the way health care is delivered, the challenge is to apply theory to practice. When a defect in the manufacture of a car model is identified, the company can recall those cars for correction, at no expense to the consumer. And on rare occasions, patient readmissions can be perceived as recalls. For example, when a department of health (DOH) assesses that the spread of an infection is due to a physician in a private office or in a hospital not meeting protocols, the DOH will require the health provider to recall all patients associated with the procedure to make sure that the break in protocol did not result in harm to many patients. But health care professionals cannot recall all patients whose care was imperfect, substandard, or inappropriate to the hospital. We need to commit to processes and methods that identify and eliminate poor care if we are to enhance the safety of patients in our health care organizations.

This book is divided into two parts. Part One, Chapters One through Four, introduces basic principles of quality management in health care and describes how health care is changing because of the public reporting of quality measures. Part Two, Chapters Five to Nine, offers the business case, explaining how quality care improves the value of health care services for the patient and for the organization. Each chapter of the book offers examples of health care issues and outlines processes for improvements. These examples, although hypothetical, are based on actual events and incorporate real responses. Each chapter ends with a summary, a list of key terms, and a set of questions called "Things to Think About."

In Chapter One I present the key drivers for changing health care practices in order to improve care and services: some drivers are external to the hospital, such as governmental agencies and private organizations, and some are internal, such as the governance, leadership, and quality management functions.

Chapter Two explains the relationship between quality data and patient safety and also the role of quality measurements in monitoring and improving health care. This chapter also outlines information on how to collect data and present the results of data analysis.

Chapter Three introduces the advantages of establishing a patient-centered environment of care. I discuss strategies to improve communication and the barriers to effective communication. The importance of patient education is also explained.

Chapter Four addresses the links among good processes and outcomes and reduced costs. Improving quality processes results in improved outcomes and reduced waste for the financial benefit of the organization. I also describe the roles of the administrative leaders, the clinicians, and quality management processes and data in improving outcomes.

In Chapter Five I discuss the value of promoting prevention to improve outcomes and reduce costs for health care organizations. Barriers to successful implementation of preventive strategies and possible ways to overcome the barriers are outlined. The roles of the government, the patient, the organization, measures, and methodologies are also discussed. I also describe problems that keep people from accepting prevention methods in the ambulatory setting and present examples of successful interventions.

In Chapter Six the high price paid by organizations and clinicians when a sentinel event occurs is reviewed. Developing processes that mitigate potential risks is not only important for patient safety but also cost effective. Once a sentinel event occurs, steps are required to correct whatever faulty processes are identified as contributing to the event.

In Chapter Seven I discuss the cost effectiveness of appropriate use of high-risk environments such as ICUs, operating rooms, and emergency departments, focusing on the advantages of establishing objective criteria for patient admission to these units and understanding the complex barriers involved in optimal utilization. I also discuss the interaction among the issues of quality of care, organizational efficiency, and financial costs when treating patients at the end of life.

Chapter Eight discusses the role of effective communication in improving patient outcomes and the importance of trust among the different levels of staff. Issues involved in reporting or not reporting poor outcomes are explained. Several examples of performance improvement efforts are offered as illustrations of using quality data and open communication to help sustain changed practices. This chapter also explains assessing staff competency through objective measures.

Chapter Nine presents issues related to promoting safety in the environment. I explain how the environment interacts with clinical care and discuss the importance of integrating safety officers and engineers into the health care team. Disaster preparedness involves not only hospital services but connections to the community and regional agencies as well.

Chapter Ten, the conclusion, reviews the points made for employing quality management processes to monitor care and define value for the patient and the organization.

PART

1

BASIC PRINCIPLES OF QUALITY MANAGEMENT

CHAPTER

1

DRIVERS OF CHANGE

LEARNING OBJECTIVES

- Identify and describe the role of external drivers of quality improvements
- Identify and describe the role of internal drivers of quality improvements
- Understand the role of quality data and measurements in monitoring care
- Describe the link between quality care and financial rewards
- Explain the role of quality management in improving patient safety

There can be no quality control or performance improvement—no way to assess safety and value—without relying on objective data about the delivery of care. Data are becoming the common language used by those involved with health care to measure quality of care and successful processes and outcomes. With data, claims of providing "good" or "excellent" care have some reality; without data, such claims are simply rhetorical.

Data that revealed that almost 100,000 people die unnecessarily in hospitals every year have helped to focus the nation's attention on medical mistakes and patient safety. Because there is so much information about the poor quality of care delivered in our hospitals, many forces outside the hospitals themselves, what I call external drivers of quality, have found it necessary to impose standards of safety and to link those standards to financial success in order to influence changes in hospital culture. These external drivers include governmental and regulatory agencies, professional medical organizations, insurers, the media, and the community (see Figure 1.1).

External drivers are working to change health care because many health care chief executive officers and chief financial officers (CEOs and CFOs) do not perceive quality outcomes and patient safety to be forces that shape a health care organization's budget. However, each of these key drivers is influencing hospital care by linking quality to finance, and together their interactive efforts have become a force for change, especially in the areas of value-based purchasing and of waste. As economic forces shape market share and hospitals compete for patients, external pressure is helping to link quality and safety to financial success.

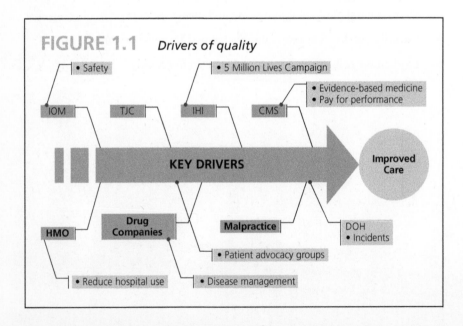

FIGURE 1.1 *Drivers of quality*

EXTERNAL DRIVERS

Leapfrog

The Leapfrog Group is an example of an organization determined to improve health care services and provide value for the health care consumer by monitoring safety and efficiency. Leapfrog was formed by a number of large corporations (General Motors, IBM, Sprint, and Toyota, among others) and agencies that purchase health care for their employees or are otherwise involved in the quality of health care. Due to their purchasing power these organizations wield a great deal of financial clout. Leapfrog attempts to influence quality and safety by rewarding those hospitals that meet certain safety standards. The idea is to force health care safety practices to "leap" forward to improve the delivery of care.

The Leapfrog Group collects data and ranks hospitals according to safety and quality standards developed by expert consultants; the data are published on the group's Web site to supply consumers of health care (including Leapfrog members' employees) with comparative information, much as *Consumer Reports* does, so they can be more informed in their choices. For example, Leapfrog recommends that employees choose hospitals that meet four standards proven to reduce the risk of error and to increase competent care:

- The hospital uses a computerized system to monitor medications, tests, and procedures. These systems reduce risks in the complex process of medication administration.

- The hospital's intensive care unit (ICU) is staffed with a full-time specialist (an intensivist). Having a full-time gatekeeper reduces risk by more clearly determining who is in charge of the patient.

- The hospital has experience with high-risk procedures. Increased experience promotes standardization and decreases variations that lead to errors.

- The hospital has a high Leapfrog safe practices score. This score reflects adherence to twenty-seven procedures ("safe practices") that the National Quality Forum and the Agency for Healthcare Research and Quality have endorsed as reducing or preventing medical errors.

In addition to promoting improved safety practices and reducing medical mistakes, the Leapfrog Group encourages transparency, the public reporting of quality and outcome measures. Those hospitals that report their outcomes score higher than those that do not. Those hospitals that comply with the Leapfrog goals often receive additional funding from insurance companies. By offering financial incentives to those hospitals that document quality, safety, and economic efficiencies, this powerful organization hopes to improve health care.

Insurers

Other private organizations are also taking it upon themselves to influence the way health care services are delivered. For example, the Health Insurance Plan of New York (HIP) is one of the largest insurers in the nation. HIP is giving bonuses to those physicians who meet specified criteria for effective communication and the delivery of compassionate care, as revealed through patient satisfaction surveys.

HIP is also collaborating with other health insurers to encourage the implementation and reporting of the Leapfrog measures, and it identifies those hospitals that participate in these activities in the HIP provider directory. Other major insurers, such as Blue Cross Blue Shield, are also developing patient safety programs and enlisting hospitals to participate and to report data on key quality and safety indicators. These insurers are conforming to the Centers for Medicare and Medicaid Services CMS position that insurers should reward good performance and refuse to reimburse poor performance.

Centers for Medicare and Medicaid Services

The Centers for Medicare and Medicaid Services, the agency that administers Medicare and Medicaid and reimburses hospitals for care expenses for patients in these programs, is in a unique position to mandate that hospitals follow specified safety standards. CMS has developed a set of initiatives, such as the pay-for-performance initiative, based on data, to track and trend medical errors. Rather than rely on physicians to report and review *adverse events*, the Office of Inspector General for the U.S. Department of Health and Human Services (HHS) reviews documentation in medical records to gather information about the delivery of care. This oversight protects the integrity of HHS programs (such as those administered by CMS) as well as the health and welfare of those served by these programs.

CMS, in partnership with other organizations, such as the National Quality Forum (NQF), the Centers for Disease Control and Prevention, the Food and Drug Administration, and the Agency for Healthcare Research and Quality, has compiled a list of adverse events related to medication errors, hospital-acquired pressure injuries, hospital-acquired infections, patient falls, and postoperative complications, that it has labeled *never events*. Data on never

ADVERSE EVENT   An adverse event is harm that is the direct result of patient–health care services interaction, not disease. The harm is caused by errors and mistakes. Such harm includes any medical error that results in death, is life threatening, requires inpatient hospitalization or prolongs hospitalization, or results in persistent or significant disability or incapacity.

NEVER EVENT A never event is a serious or life-endangering medical error, such as surgery on the wrong patient. The National Quality Forum (NQF) deems such events to be ones that should never occur in a health care setting. In collaboration with consumers, providers, purchasers, researchers, and other health care stakeholders, the NQF has defined twenty-eight of these preventable errors that health care organizations are expected to report and take steps to correct. (See Chapter Six.)

events are reported to the public. Hospitals that show a lack of compliance with safety indicators for never events might face economic consequences, such as lack of payment.

CMS has also established a quality incentive initiative, pay for performance, offering participating hospitals whose data show that they are in the top decile of all hospitals that report compliance with standardized quality measures a 2 percent bonus on their Medicare payments. Hospitals in the second decile will receive a 1 percent bonus. In other words, hospitals will get paid for delivering good care.

The goal is to improve the quality and value of health care and to change the way care is delivered. Rigorous studies and research have concluded that certain factors have a positive impact on patient outcomes. The application of these factors to care is known as *evidence-based medicine*, and it is evidence-based medicine that is the basis of the pay-for-performance indicators. By financially rewarding organizations that can prove they are delivering quality care, the government is hoping to encourage changed practices, especially in the management of chronic diseases such as heart failure and pneumonia.

State Departments of Health

Departments of health (DOHs) at the state level are also attempting to change the delivery of health care, making it safer and more efficient—and less costly—by promoting transparency. For example, the New York State DOH Web site provides information to potential health care consumers about

RISK-ADJUSTED DATA The intent of risk adjusting is to make fair comparisons among patients across organizations. Risk adjustment is a statistical process that allows one to understand and compensate for data set variations that would otherwise prevent accurate comparison. By applying a formula, risk adjusters can identify patients with different risk factors that might affect their outcomes.

EVIDENCE-BASED MEDICINE Evidence-based medicine is the gold standard of care. Recommendations for treatment of specific diseases are based on expert advice about best practices, the most comprehensive and up-to-date research, and the results of clinical trials. Evidence-based medicine is the alternative to the isolated decisions of independent practitioners; it gathers knowledge and experience from the members of the medical community and then provides cumulative knowledge and experience back to the entire medical community.

physicians, hospitals, nursing homes, patient complaints, and cardiac surgery mortality rates. The rationale behind the transparency movement is to provide the buying public with information about health care choices. New York State publishes brochures explaining the *risk-adjusted* data in lay language, hoping to dispel some of the mystique that surrounds clinical phenomena such as cardiac bypass surgery. With accessible health care information, consumers can take responsibility for choosing where they want to go to be treated and hospitals can compete for market share by improving processes.

Joint Commission

The Joint Commission is an independent, not-for-profit organization that evaluates hospitals for accreditation by examining how well they meet specified standards designed to reduce risk to patients and ensure organizational accountability and efficiency. Without accreditation, hospitals do not receive Medicare reimbursements. Therefore hospitals that are not accredited will suffer financially. More than half of the Joint Commission standards are related to patient safety; Joint Commission surveyors expect hospitals to review data about medication, infection, transfusions, staff competence, fire safety, medical equipment, and many other factors.

The Joint Commission also requires that adverse events be reported and corrected and that organizations take steps to prevent harm by identifying vulnerable processes. It champions transparency of information about

SENTINEL EVENT Sentinel event is a term used by the Joint Commission to describe an unanticipated or unexpected medical error that results in serious physical or psychological consequences for the patient. The Joint Commission tracks such events in a database, with the intent of alerting health care organizations to problems leading to such events and of promoting preventive measures to avoid these problems.

quality and cost and has been in the forefront of changing the hospital culture so that patients are informed about bad outcomes. *Sentinel events* are tracked by the Joint Commission, and data relating to underlying causes, as defined through root cause analysis (see Chapters Two and Six), are published and shared with the nation's health care organizations. National Patient Safety Goals (see Chapter Five) have been defined by the Joint Commission, which assesses how organizations attempt to meet these goals during the accreditation review.

Institute for Healthcare Improvement

The Institute for Healthcare Improvement (IHI) is another agency that has brought the risks of hospitalization to public attention. Its initial Saving Lives campaign was a national effort to reduce medical errors that resulted in unnecessary death for 100,000 people. The goal of that campaign was to highlight awareness of patient safety and to encourage hospitals to voluntarily report data about improved processes and to share best practices on both regional and national levels. A new initiative, the 5 Million Lives Campaign, intended to prevent 5 million incidents of medical harm over a two-year period, was launched in December 2006. The IHI has defined twelve changes in care that would reduce patient harm, from preventing surgical site infections through appropriate antibiotic use to getting the board on board to improve oversight of patient safety. The IHI goal is that hospital governing boards should spend more than 25 percent of their meeting time on quality and safety issues.

Other Drivers

In addition to the organizations already discussed, many other agencies are monitoring quality standards and holding hospitals accountable for providing data about quality care. These organizations include the National Quality Forum (NQF), a group of public and private organizations working to promote measures of health care quality and improvement; the National Patient Safety Foundation (NPSF), an organization of health care professionals committed to making patient safety a national priority; and the Agency for Healthcare Research and Quality (AHRQ), the research arm of the Department of Health and Human Services, which is charged with improving safety and reducing the costs of health care services. The AHRQ supports research on evidence-based outcomes, quality, and cost.

These and other external drivers of quality, from governmental, business, insurance, and consumer groups, are changing medical culture, making the specifics of the delivery of services available to the public. Physicians can no longer hide, as they once might have, behind a wall of specialized language. This move toward transparency allows patients to understand the risks and benefits of any procedure.

The Public

The public eye has also become a force for change. The pledge to "do no harm" is no longer sufficient as a description of what patients want. That is the least of it. They don't want to be struck with an antibiotic-resistant infection because a health care worker has not washed his or her hands. They certainly don't want to have a wrong-site surgery or to be transfused with the wrong blood or to be administered incorrect medication or to fall. Public awareness is forcing health care institutions to maintain a high standard of quality or risk failing financially. Hospitals have to provide information to the public that details what value is exchanged for people's health care spending.

Hospitals that participate in the national safety agenda and are willing to promote transparency have data about their provision of care published on Web sites that are available to the public. Leaders at these hospitals want the community to trust that the services at their hospitals are safe and reliable; not participating in these initiatives might be seen as suspect by the public.

Increased transparency regarding processes and problems encourages organizations to do proactive analyses of gaps in care, with the goal of discovering vulnerable areas in the care process. For example, the staph infection MRSA (methicillin resistant *Staphylococcus aureus*) has been in the news lately because it is drug resistant and rampant and is infecting and even killing people. By performing a root cause analysis (see Chapter Six), organizations can identify which patients have become infected and trace the source of the infection. Infection control specialists trained in epidemiology can recommend preventive actions to the medical board, such as clustering patients with infections in one area so that the infection doesn't spread.

The New York State Committee to Reduce Infection Deaths recommends steps that a patient should take to protect against infection. One recommendation is to choose a surgeon with a low infection rate; such rates are now available to the public. The more information a patient has, the better care that patient will receive. Patients are encouraged to take a proactive role, reminding caregivers to wash their hands, requesting antibiotics prophylactically before surgery, reminding doctors to monitor glucose levels, and avoiding urinary catheters if possible.

Today, patients are encouraged to intervene for their own safety. Although this burdens the patient, other interventions have not been successful. Some hospitals have assigned nurses to watch each physician and remind him or her to wash his or her hands. Others have installed cameras to view which staff comply with hand-washing requirements and which do not. I know of one organization that rewarded doctors who washed their hands with superior parking lot spaces. Most of these ideas are doomed to failure in the long run because they are not really about health or the patient, nor are they intrinsic to the clinician.

It's extraordinary that in today's world lack of proper hand washing is the number one reason that patients become infected and that therefore poor hand hygiene represents the greatest danger to patient safety. What prevents care-givers from washing their hands? Culture. Hand hygiene is perhaps not technical enough or medical enough or interesting enough to be taken seri-ously as a threat to health. If it were internalized that poor hand hygiene kills people, perhaps habits would change. Such an enculturation requires reeduca-tion of staff and leadership commitment.

When patients are too ill to monitor their care, it behooves their families and loved ones to take charge and ensure that appropriate care is provided. When my son needed hand surgery, the surgeon explained that there was a 5 percent chance of infection and that such a rate was normal. Not for me. I left and found a surgeon who explained to me what precautions he took to have zero infections after surgery. Happily it was not an emergency situation, and I could afford the time to choose the best physician. My son couldn't do it, but I could. Family members should become active when patients themselves are unable to.

INTERNAL DRIVERS

The governmental and public movement to oversee the quality of care deliv-ered in hospitals has come about in part because of the lack of oversight within hospitals. Physicians do not set standards of care for other physicians, nor do they monitor the treatment and outcome results of other physicians. If there is a poor outcome or an adverse event, the state department of health usually gets involved to review a particular physician's file and assess com-petency. Professional conduct committees are established for peer reviews. If it is determined that the physician delivered substandard care, action is taken, from suspending a license to delivering a rebuke to requiring reeducation.

However, there is no watchdog group internal to the hospital or health care organization to oversee, monitor, evaluate, and take action. The watch-dog should be a quality management department (QMD), an objective entity that reports to the governance and the CEO. The QMD can focus on standards of care without being influenced by particular interest groups. Unfortunately, such a role is rarely assigned to a QMD because many administrators believe that the board should not be involved in "running the hospital."

Getting the Board on Board

Health care reformers realize that unless the governing board gets on board with the national safety agenda to improve the delivery of care, there is little chance of success or change in any health care organization. Traditionally, the governing board was responsible for the financial health of the organization; today its role has evolved to include oversight of patient safety and efficient and effective organizational processes.

In order for board members to understand the specifics of the clinical care they are charged to oversee, they have to be educated—by clinicians and by quality professionals. They need to have training in interpreting data as these data are presented to them, and they need to learn how to ask focused questions about poor outcomes. Primarily, they need to believe that medicine is neither magical nor too specialized for lay understanding.

To do their job, board members should insist on clear presentations of data and explanations and interpretations of data that enable them to evaluate care and processes for improvement. They need to understand their organization's numbers and what they mean, and how these numbers compare to national numbers. They also need to define for themselves their goals for patient care: how much infection can be tolerated as "normal"? What rate of surgical mortality is acceptable? What rate of pressure injuries is reasonable? The board can help the organization with defining its priorities and its philosophy of care.

Board members also need to be able to distinguish "good" care from "bad" and "excellent" from "acceptable." These are value-laden terms. What exactly is meant by being the "best"? How is "best" defined? Board members need to be educated about quality indicators, quality data, and comparative analysis. They should also become familiar with analytical techniques, such as root cause analysis and failure mode and effects analysis (see Chapter Three). They are the eyes, ears, and voice of the community. They watch, they listen, and they need to let the organization know the direction in which to move.

The board of trustees, sitting at the top of the chain of accountability, by asking simple questions and by demanding coherent explanations rather than easy rationalizations, can increase the value of health care delivery. If the board asks clinicians to explain why people are dying, it expects the clinician to offer a better answer than that the patients are very sick. If the patients are dying from complications of surgery, board members want to know what the complications are, what causes them, how they can be avoided, and what the medical board is doing about improving the situation. If the board wants to know whether the ICU is being used to house terminal patients who get no benefit from high-tech treatment and, if so, why those patients are not in a palliative care setting, physicians should be prepared to explain. And if the explanations are not satisfactory, changes should be made.

Quality management professionals can help train board members to interpret data and ask effective questions of administrative and clinical leaders. Through education and with information, board members can quickly become competent to evaluate care and to recognize gaps in patient safety that require repair. No one is suggesting that board members perform surgery, only that they ask why an unnecessary complication, such as infection, occurs after surgery.

FIGURE 1.2 *Executive summary: Patient safety indicators*

Example	2006	2007	
Nosocomial pressure ulcer rate	1.01	1.06	⬤
Patient fall index	3.75	2.82	▼
Patient medical and surgical restraint index	28.58	43.85	◆

◆	Increasing rate or average - statistically significant performance decline
⬤	Statistically no significant change
▼	Decreasing rate or average - statistically significant improvement

I have taught board members the fundamentals of measurement and root cause analysis, the requirements of corrective actions, the importance of compliance with evidence-based quality indicators, and the rationale behind the regulatory and governmental push for improved patient safety. Board members are pleased to gain the tools to do their jobs effectively.

Quality management staff should use data reports to educate the board about progress and problems in the delivery of care. Especially when tracked and trended over time and when compared to other institutions and against national benchmarks, measures of care can be effectively monitored.

Figure 1.2 is an example of an effective graphic representation of how a hospital is performing on specific patient safety indicators. These particular indicators are classified as never events. If the hospital were improving safety practices, each measure would be lower than it was the previous year. When presented with quality information in this format, a board member can quickly assess which areas require further improvement and which areas have successfully improved.

Enlisting the C Suite

Adopting the business model of referring to the CEO, COO (chief operating officer), CMO (chief medical officer), and CFO as the "C suite" focuses attention on their roles as executives responsible for successful business practices and results. The product that their business is producing is medical care, and a good product is defined as good outcomes that result from efficient, effective, and safe care. The C suite represents the primary drivers of quality that are internal to a hospital or health care organization.

The chief medical officer provides the primary leadership for the clinicians. Together with the medical board of the hospital, the CMO sets standards of care and defines best practices. The Joint Commission defines the role that the medical board has in overseeing clinical quality. Medical board members evaluate clinical and technical competency through the credentialing and recredentialing process and determine appropriate treatment interventions. Included in their oversight responsibilities are evaluating surgical performance, approving new procedures, and analyzing new medications and adverse drug reactions, as well as evaluating the efficacy and cost of comparable drugs. (If the generic brand has the same efficacy and is less expensive, the medical board can suggest using it.) They review infection rates, infection sources, and interventions to reduce infections. They examine trends and target improvement efforts. They look at mortality rates, by diagnosis, disease, and complication, and try to provide education about appropriate care delivery. In sum, the medical board is responsible for every aspect of clinical care. Therefore, if the members take their role seriously and do their job effectively, they are the primary internal drivers of quality.

By joining forces, the board of trustees, the C suite, and the medical board can provide value to the patients and to the health care organization they lead. The quality management department supports the activities of the medical board by providing ongoing data analysis, tracking and trending outcomes, identifying gaps in patient safety, and defining best practices. Quality management can also help to educate the board and leadership in understanding public report cards and providing valid and accurate data to national groups. Together these groups set standards for quality. There is no way to understand the provision of care for 100 or 1,000 or 10,000 patients without an objective process analysis based on data.

When adverse events occur, quality management staff typically help clinicians to prepare their presentation of the occurrence to the medical board and also, if necessary, to the appropriate state or regulatory agency. The physician and quality management staff develop corrective actions which the medical board is expected to approve. If the adverse event requires a peer review to ascertain competency, the medical board assigns either internal or external physicians to review the case.

But many medical boards do not accept these responsibilities. Many physicians are not aware that they need to report an event—even when there has been no serious harm to the patient. Typically, they fix the problem and move on. However, if this gap in care is not identified, most likely it will happen again and a patient could indeed be harmed. Many physicians do not realize that they have the responsibility to monitor quality of care or to establish standards.

With the push to transparency, there is no choice but to define measures, collect data, and be prepared to explain why the data show that care is not 100 percent optimal. If physicians dismiss the data as flawed, that makes little difference to an indignant public, who will be informed if one hospital's mortality rate is higher than the national average, for example, or if its infection rate is higher than the rate at a neighboring hospital. Rather than argue about the data, the medical board needs to institute improvements and let the public see improved results.

Every clinician should be informed about gaps and improvement efforts. When the medical board has information to deliver, communication to the medical staff can take place via grand rounds. In fact the Joint Commission has made effective communication among physicians a focus for continuing medical education (CME) credit. Improving procedures is part of medical education.

The medical board, the board of trustees, and the quality management department share responsibility for value, for providing safe care and efficient services with reductions in cost. For example, if data show that many patients require a specialized diet, the medical board, nutritional services, and quality management should develop policies and procedures, and also measures to monitor and evaluate the results of the procedures. Good processes result in improved outcomes. Constant feedback should be part of a deliberate improvement process; the Plan-Do-Check-Act (PDCA) cycle (see Chapter Four), for instance, is used by many industries to change processes and improve. Caregivers must communicate effectively for care to be efficient. For example, clinicians often overlook nutrition as an important medical intervention. But of course it is one. The dietician and those responsible for the delivery of food have to work collaboratively with the clinicians to ensure safe and efficient care.

Just think about it. If a patient is scheduled for surgery and there is no process to include dietary services in the information loop and the patient has food delivered because of this communication failure, that patient's surgery has to be postponed. If the operating room schedule is interrupted, the result is waste—poor value. If a patient who is diabetic or who has heart failure is fed an improper diet, the result can be a longer length of stay (LOS) and complications. The hospital loses money on each inappropriately long LOS—poor value. When care and services are in separate silos, a situation marked by a lack of coordination and communication, this pattern has to be changed to ensure safe and efficient services.

Driving Change with Quality Data

Quality control and performance improvement, safety, and value rely on objective data about the delivery of care. Everyone working in a health care environment, from the frontline caregivers to the members of the hospital's board of trustees, should understand the value of data and become familiar with the basics of quality management. Data shape the definition of quality care as the outcome of appropriate interventions based on statistical evidence and the identification of best practices.

Most organizations do not school their staff on the basics of using data for defining quality care. This is unfortunate, because there is no better way to prove that outcomes are good (with low complication rates and quick recovery rates, for example) and processes are efficient and effective (so that they reduce waste by minimizing reoperation and readmission, for example). Data are critical not only for defining excellence but also for targeting opportunities for improvements. If staff are taught to use data to identify which processes require improvements, which processes are vulnerable to failure and to errors, where the gaps are in patient safety, and how efficiently resources are being used, the organization can make improvements.

With accurate and explanatory data, decision makers can make informed decisions about patient safety, resource management, and financial allocation. With the appropriate use of data, patients are safer and money is spent most effectively. Therefore, learning how to define measurements that formulate the data, creating databases to aggregate and analyze the data, and communicating the results of analysis effectively to the relevant people in the organization requires a conscious and deliberate process—as well as an understanding of the fundamental value of measures.

Driving Safety with Quality Management

A quality management department that employs a methodology can objectively and proactively evaluate care to sustain improvements over time and create a patient-focused culture of quality and safety. Such a department relies on the social sciences to explain structure, process, function, and roles, especially in communicating a problem identified as contributing to a poor outcome. Quality management processes rely on operational research to reduce defects in the delivery of care, incorporating the entire caregiving team, not only the primary physician.

As long as there have been healers of the sick, the idea of good care, or quality care, has been difficult to define. From the classical "do no harm" to Florence Nightingale's pioneering work linking disease and treatment to the modern push for transparency with the public reporting of quality indicators, the public has looked for assurance from the medical community that patients will be safe.

People seek such assurance not only from the physicians who treat them but from the larger health care organization as well. Ernest A. Codman, a physician champion of quality in the early 1900s, was among the first to suggest that hospitals be held responsible for explaining, understanding, and improving poor outcomes. He took the unpopular position that the health care organization was accountable for providing quality care, and that if patients were harmed and outcomes were poor, the organization should attempt to discover the reason and institute improvements. Codman realized that poor outcomes were often the result of a confluence of factors, many of them small or subtle mistakes in processes that eventually added up to a bigger problem. His notion was that by analyzing poor outcomes, future failures might be prevented.

Codman also believed in transparency in health care, long before it became a buzzword in the modern discourse about patient safety. He wanted to remove the veil of mystery that shrouded health care outcomes. He wanted the public to be informed so that they could make informed choices about where they wanted to be treated. His innovative ideas moved the concept of quality from process evaluation (asking whether a certain procedure was done or not done) to linking processes with outcomes or end results (asking whether the procedure resulted in good or bad outcomes).

Today, health care leaders recognize that quality care is defined along three dimensions: using evidence-based medicine as the standard of care, documenting that that standard has been met by the organization, and monitoring data extracted from documentation and other sources of information about processes and outcomes for various patient populations. These three dimensions provide the quality management department with the tools needed to evaluate the delivery of care.

Using Quality Data

Quality management is more than quality control or quality improvement or a method to comply with regulatory requirements. Quality management's objectives are to assess care, to identify problems and best practices, and to promote improvements, and all these actions require objective criteria—in short, data. Data are impersonal. Data can provide the definitions of good care and of poor outcomes.

Many businesses and organizations make use of quality data and measurements to enhance their performance and improve their profits. For some reason, health care has been slow to understand that it is a business and as such could benefit from good business practices. As with any business, positive publicity about good results brings increased market share; in the case of health care, good results bring patients into hospitals, whereas poor reports drive them elsewhere. Many physicians do not believe that poor hospital report cards can hurt their relationship with their patients. However, the cumulative experiences of the physician influence the survival of the hospital.

Decision makers have to become adept at understanding variables that relate quality, cost, resource utilization, waste, and satisfaction in order to provide value to the community of patients. Data should be used by leadership to understand factors that increase or decrease the use of expensive resources. Lowering costs and maximizing efficiency is good business and improves profits. There is no way to monitor care and cost without data.

For example, the reengineering movement was an administrative attempt to use efficiency models to change and improve hospital care. It did not work for many reasons, among them that the model was focused on budgetary concerns and had little regard for the clinical information required to understand the delivery of good care. Cost savings made without regard to quality information generally end up backfiring; they eventually require extra and unnecessary expenditures to repair problems arising from complications, maloccurrences, adverse events, poor publicity, organizational disruptions, and so on. The reengineering solution of reducing cost by redesigning the work flow that led to reducing nursing staff had a negative impact on clinical outcomes. The focus was on replacing nursing with a less expensive workforce rather than on providing quality care.

To ensure that quality of care is preserved while finances are reduced, quality data should be merged with financial data to appropriately evaluate resource priorities. Leaders should receive information about

- Clinical variables that indicate waste, such as reoperation rates, waiting times in the emergency department, and turnaround times in the operating room

- Overuse of hospital beds

- Clinical variables that indicate quality of care, such as infection rates, incident rates, complication rates, mortality rates, admission to the ICU postoperatively, and end-of-life measures

- Outcome indicators by disease, benchmarked against CMS measures

These variables, along with financial indicators, enable decision makers to understand the complex interactions involved in the delivery of quality care.

The Joint Commission supports data collection and analysis because these activities lead to improved care. The Joint Commission requires documentation about important aspects of care (such as infection rates and blood utilization), organizational management, and the environment of care. With established measurements, consistent standards of care can be defined, patient safety can be monitored, and improvements can be assessed over time. In order to receive accreditation, hospitals must be surveyed by the Joint Commission, which expects them to be able to prove that they are complying with quality standards. The proof is in the data and in their use. Data should be used to target and monitor improvements.

Health care leaders are beginning to realize that explanations of medical phenomena are not found by asking individual physicians about an individual patient's situation. Rather, medical care is better explained by analyzing aggregated data about patient populations. For example, how many patients over seventy-five years old were admitted with pneumonia during a specific time frame? How many pneumonia patients received education regarding vaccination before discharge? On what day after admission were pneumonia patients switched to oral antibiotics? What was the average LOS for pneumonia patients? Policies should be based on these kinds of data and improvement efforts prioritized on the basis of those data.

Another example involves analysis of errors. The medical community agrees that no patient should have surgery on the wrong site. Wrong-site surgery is considered a sentinel event by the Joint Commission. If the data reported to the organizational leadership reveal zero events of wrong-site

EXAMPLE: SUICIDE

A sentinel event tends to draw the CEO's attention. However, it is generally looked on as a rare and random accident, rather than as a predictable result of faulty processes. Consider what happens when there is a suicide (which the Joint Commission names the second most prevalent sentinel event in hospitals). The CEO will get all kinds of assurances that this event was entirely unpredictable and one that fortunately occurs very rarely. However, if the event is analyzed in terms of what defects in care enabled the patient to come to harm, the CEO and others in decision-making roles will be able to determine the difference between a random accident and a broken process. Once the gaps in the process of care are revealed, steps can be taken to improve.

When my quality management department wanted to understand just such an event at one of the acute care hospitals in our health care system, we began to collect data on how many suicides and attempted suicides had occurred on medical units in our system over a period of years. The medical records of the relevant patients were examined. For every suicide event, two schematics were developed in the form of flow charts, one detailing what had actually occurred and a second outlining what should have happened to preserve the patient's safety. Analysis revealed that almost 12 percent of these medical patients had the comorbidity of alcoholism, a syndrome well known to be associated with an increased risk of suicide. Further analysis revealed that when these patients were initially assessed, their alcoholism was not diagnosed. Had it been, these patients might have received medication to prevent the progression of withdrawal symptoms, symptoms that were found to be implicated in acute care suicide.

The result of a three-year patient safety initiative was changed protocols and new tools for diagnosis of vulnerable patients entering the hospital through the emergency department for medical problems. Had the rare event been dismissed as a tragic accident and never analyzed, important improvements would not have resulted.

surgery, care is good. However, if the data show that wrong-site surgery has occurred, the care is considered substandard. The reason for the problem has to be identified and analyzed, new processes have to be introduced to improve performance, and the improvement efforts have to be monitored over time. When appropriately analyzed and presented coherently, data can be a force to change behavior.

SUMMARY

Hospitals are changing the way care is delivered due to

- Pressure from governmental and regulatory agencies to improve care

- Increased transparency, such as public reports of quality variables and outcome measures

- The introduction of financial consequences for poor quality

- Media exposure of risks to patient safety in hospital care

- Increased governance and leadership accountability for good outcomes

 ## KEY TERMS

CMS
drivers of quality
evidence-based medicine
Joint Commission

pay for performance
public report cards
quality management
transparency

 ## THINGS TO THINK ABOUT

Imagine that you have just been hired to oversee quality at a multihospital health care system. Your initial goal is to do a cost-benefit analysis of the quality processes in the organization.

1. Which personnel and staff will you contact to assess the quality of care?

2. Whom would you target to be accountable for the quality process?

3. How would you oversee compliance versus improvements?

4. How would you evaluate adding resources to the quality of care?

CHAPTER

2

IMPROVING PATIENT SAFETY

LEARNING OBJECTIVES

- Describe how data can be used to define *good* care for physicians and administrators; explain how quality measures can be used to define value

- Describe the link between quality care and organizational efficiency

- Understand the role of root cause analysis in defining gaps to patient safety

- Identify appropriate formats for data analysis reports

Administrators and physicians have been somewhat reluctant to get on the quality data bandwagon, but there simply is no other way to assess or improve patient safety. The reasons for their reluctance provoke interesting questions about the delivery of care. Usually, these reasons involve hospital culture, a term that refers to entrenched habits of mind and behavior. Administrators typically adhere to a culture in which physician practice is not questioned by nonphysicians. The traditional division between the financial and administrative end of the organization and the clinical practice is well established. Physicians typically adhere to a culture of independence and self-reliance. They are trained to address individual and unique conditions and tailor treatment to specific patients. They are not familiar with using aggregated data about patient populations (other than data from clinical trials) or accepting recommendations for treatment from governmental agencies or medical societies.

Convincing administrative and clinical leadership and staff that their administrative and medical decisions should be data driven requires focused education. Administrators become convinced of the usefulness and value of quality data when confronted with the obvious link between good care and profit. Good care is not due to chance but is the result of deliberate processes that focus on good outcomes. Good care is defined and explained through data, data that show few adverse outcomes, reduced infection rates, low complication rates, reduced falls, few pressure injuries, and increased patient volume and satisfaction. Good care also reduces resource consumption—data show increased bed turnover rates, efficient processes that diminish unnecessary expenses, and few malpractice suits. Not a hard sell, right? Yet administrators have to be educated about the link between quality and finance.

For physicians, accepting compliance with quality measures is more difficult because their autonomy in deciding treatment has been sacrosanct. But physicians, as scientists, respond to proof and when shown objective data that their practices result in outcomes that are poorer than the outcomes of others in their organization, region, state, or nation, they take notice. For example, if data reveal that orthopedic patients coming to one hospital for joint replacements have zero complications and data also reveal that a similar patient population having the same procedure in a comparable hospital does have complications, a longer hospital stay, and poorer levels of function when released, physicians at the second hospital will begin to think about what they are doing incorrectly and will ask for more data and analysis to reevaluate their processes and make changes. The objectivity of data helps to diminish outcries of bias or personal agendas.

Cultural change is required to improve care and enhance the value of changing the delivery of care. Cultural change is focused on the physician as a member of the care delivery team, the leader who determines the treatment and supervises the care through the delegation of responsibilities to others. Medical leadership needs to support cultural change through data. With the help of quality management professionals, the medical staff should be introduced to statistical data and given the ability to analyze results to explain problems that prevent recovery, to reveal poor communication, to detail variation from the standard of care, and to identify organizational bottlenecks that harm the patient and waste the hospital's resources. Cultural change is also required to instill new attitudes toward documentation, especially a habit of using the medical record to effectively communicate the treatment plan to all caregivers.

UNDERSTANDING QUALITY MEASURES

Because it is so obvious that care cannot be monitored or improved without data, organizations are pressured to use data to establish *quality indicators* to be collected and reported to external organizations such as the Centers for Medicare and Medicaid Services (CMS) and the Institute for Healthcare Improvement (IHI).

Through data these agencies plan to drive quality care processes to improve. Using data CMS will decide which health care organizations will receive financial rewards and accreditation and which will not. Like it or not, organizations now have to develop processes and assign personnel for data collection if they are to participate in the health care marketplace.

CEOs are increasingly aware of the power of quality measures to draw patients to particular hospitals. Therefore they are struggling with how best to present measures to the public. In order to maintain their competitive edge, organizations need to establish a data collection process, determine who will be accountable for collecting and reporting the data, and then develop a methodology for analyzing the data and using them to improve patient outcomes and increase patient safety.

Typically, and unfortunately, quality data generally travel directly from the quality management department to the regulatory agency, bypassing administrative and clinical leadership. Not long ago, I sat with a CFO and a vice president for managed care, discussing the *quality measures* that had to be reported in order for their hospital to receive increased reimbursement. The only topic of interest to them was how to document compliance. They were not able to see beyond the compliance issue to the intent of the measures— improving processes for improved patient outcomes. To these administrators, collecting and reporting measures were considered inconveniences, paperwork

QUALITY INDICATOR   A quality indicator is a process or outcome measure that is used to determine performance, usually an agreed-upon variable that measures adherence to a standard or to the achievement of quality.

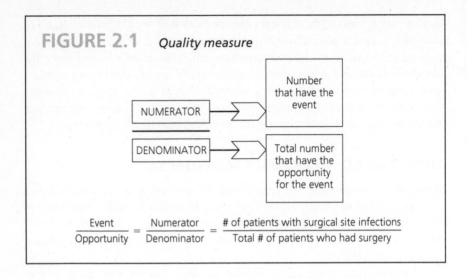

FIGURE 2.1 *Quality measure*

$$\frac{\text{Event}}{\text{Opportunity}} = \frac{\text{Numerator}}{\text{Denominator}} = \frac{\text{\# of patients with surgical site infections}}{\text{Total \# of patients who had surgery}}$$

QUALITY MEASURE

A quality measure consists of two numbers: one represents an event (or set of events) and the other represents a circumstance where there were opportunities for that event to occur. Measures are defined as the event divided by the opportunity. The event is the numerator (N) and the opportunity is the denominator (D). (See Figure 2.1.)

that had to be generated simply to meet requirements. However, when CEOs, CFOs, and other executives use quality data in the way these indicators are meant to be used, to understand processes of care and to target weak areas for improvement, it would make their jobs easier and their organization more successful financially.

For example, if you are concerned with surgical site infections, you collect data about the number of people who were diagnosed with a surgical site infection (N) during a specified time period. That's the event. The denominator is the total number of patients who had surgery during that same time period. If the data show that 100 people had surgery in a month and of those 100 people, 10 developed an infection, then the infection rate is 10 over 100 or 10 percent. If more refinement is needed, you can analyze the data further by procedure or physician.

WORKING WITH QUALITY INFORMATION

If data collection reveals an infection rate of 10 percent, what should that information mean to an administrative leader or unit manager, and what

EXAMPLE: REPORTING INFECTION RATES

A typical report on infection might look like Table 2.1. This report tracks two of the CMS measures for reducing infection: discontinuing antibiotics within twenty-four hours after surgery and administering antibiotics within one hour prior to surgery. Evidence shows that both these measures reduce infection. The report shows the rate of compliance with each measure, and also compares the rates over time, by quarter. The goal is for the rate to be above the CMS benchmark (three stars). Falling below the CMS benchmark (one star) indicates that processes should be improved. This simple scorecard is presented to the board of trustees and graphically informs board members about compliance with these measures. They can see at a glance when the goal is met and when not and can investigate why the goals are not met.

When improvement seems indicated, leaders should establish task forces, made up of professionals from all relevant disciplines, to analyze existing processes and recommend interventions that might improve those processes. Without multidisciplinary and interdepartmental communication, it is difficult to understand the big picture—what is actually happening to the patient during the episode of hospitalization and what the impact on the organization is. Teams led by infection control specialists can brainstorm data on infection and recommend preventive strategies.

In this example, the team might consist of surgeons, anesthesiologists, infection control specialists, operating room nurses, quality management staff, and research analysts. The medical staff can explain to the team how complications from infection have an impact on the patient's health and require expensive resources such as the operating room or intensive care unit (ICU). A member of the risk management department might report on how much infection costs the organization in malpractice claims and lawsuits, and someone from utilization might explain how much infection costs the organization in excess days of stay. Someone in public relations might explore how poor publicity about the infection rate has had an impact on the volume of patients. All too often in hospitals, people in one department do not communicate with people in other departments.

The medical records of patients who acquired infections should be analyzed by the team. Once the underlying causes of the infections are identified through root cause analysis, the team should develop protocols to improve faulty processes. The team should research the available literature to adapt whatever might be useful to its organization. A tremendous amount of knowledge has already been published. Senior leaders, such as the CEO, COO, and

CFO, should be involved in the improvement effort because they need to understand the organizational implications of improving processes—professional time and additional financial outlay may be needed. Measures should be developed to track the changes in the processes, and staff designated to collect and document the data. Databases, which may be Web based, should be developed for analysts to use. Data should track the rate of change and the implementation of preventive strategies by physician, unit, division, or patient population.

Prevention provides more value than reaction. All these professionals together can help the health care organization define the value of reducing its infection rate, both for patient safety and for an improved bottom line. The two are inexorably connected.

TABLE 2.1   **HQA-CMS public reporting of surgical care infection prevention (SCIP)**

	2007 Q1	2007 Q2	2007 Q3	2007 Q4	2008 Q1	2008 Q2
SCIP prophylactic antibiotics discontinued within 24 hrs. after surgery end time: overall rate	93%	93%	96%	93%	95%	97%
	**	**	***	**	**	**
SCIP prophylactic antibiotics within 1 hr. prior to surgical incision: overall rate	96%	98%	97%	76%	89%	98%
	***	***	***	*	**	***

*** Hospital performed above the CMS top 10th percentile
** Hospital performed between the CMS 10th percentile and the 50th percentile
* Hospital performed below the CMS 50th percentile

should be done with the information? Who in the organization can best advise leadership? Who should be charged with improvements, and what kinds of improvements are reasonable and financially viable? Usually nurses collect the data and submit it to the unit manager who, if the data reveal poor care, may defensively challenge the validity of the data. Quality data should instead be sent directly to quality management for reliability testing and analysis.

Quality management professionals use objective measurements to assess the delivery of care, and research analysts trained in quality management methods are able to ensure that data are valid and to analyze valid data for trends. They are familiar with statistical analysis and have the capability to create reports that illustrate how one organization compares to other similar organizations. Quality analysts can establish **benchmarks**, or standards, for an organization to meet.

MEASURING VALUE

In order to establish value in health care, the patient has to benefit, as does the organization and the staff. Benefit is defined by measures. For example, if a surgical patient does not get a wound infection and has a short length of stay (LOS) and an early discharge, it benefits the patient and the organization— that's value. Measures can be used to describe outcomes such as surgical site infections, mortality, ventilator-associated pneumonias, days in the ICU, and reoperations. All these measures are associated with patient safety. The lower the number of complications, the greater the benefit; waste and additional work are reduced.

Other measures can be used to describe the process of care, answering questions like these; Did the patient receive medication in a timely way? Was the informed consent properly understood and signed? Were the nutritional needs of the patient correctly assessed? Was the history and physical complete? Linking measures of quality and of value enables leaders to understand how specific processes link to specific outcomes. There is a value in connecting processes with clinical outcomes or financial outcomes, or both. In the health system where I work, we developed a table of measures to inform system leadership about the delivery of care and organizational processes.

When health care leadership connects information about processes and outcomes, the connection illustrates something about the scope of the problem and the value of the solution. The value is both clinical and organizational. Clinically, a timely diagnosis might avoid unnecessary death in the emergency department (ED). Providing appropriate and timely intervention eliminates a potential risk-management issue and possible malpractice claims. Timely diagnosis also reduces crowded conditions in the ED and enables interventions that move the patient rapidly along the continuum of care. If efforts are made to increase the delivery of aspirin in a timely way and patient

EXAMPLE: ACUTE MYOCARDIAL INFARCTION

Evidence-based medicine has shown that when aspirin (among other interventions) is given within four hours of admittance to the emergency department (ED) to patients suffering from heart attack (acute myocardial infarction, or AMI), mortality is lower than it is when aspirin is not given within that time frame. That information is useful for clinicians as a clinical marker and for the establishment of order sets. The information is also useful for administrators because it reveals how accurate and timely the ED is in providing appropriate care. If AMI patients are not diagnosed and treated in a timely way, it might be due to problems related to triage, throughput, or *queuing*. Rapid responses to problems save lives and also keep the organizational processes moving without interruption. Many organizations have started to use data to evaluate processes and make recommendations for improvements.

QUEUING THEORY Queuing theory explores the relationship between random customer demands and fixed organizational capacity. In health care, queuing focuses on patient flow, attempting to maximize efficiency by avoiding delays caused by poor coordination of services, by matching staff resources to patient needs, and by continuous monitoring and tracking of patients, with links to actions.

EXAMPLE: FALLS

Data on falls, another patient safety indicator, are also required by the CMS and other regulatory organizations. Patients should not fall; when they do, there are often complications such as broken bones, infections, longer LOS, surgery, and lawsuits. Falls are measurable; prevention programs can be developed and instituted. However, fall prevention has become so much a part of the health care routine, especially now that the population is aging, with most patients on fall prevention management, that staff may be less vigilant than they should be.

Although nurses who have had the primary responsibility of preventing falls have been oriented toward preventing falls for years, patients still fall. The old processes simply are not effective. New interventions are clearly required to address this patient safety issue. In order to assess the value of the interventions, someone has to be looking at the data—and at the process. You cannot establish a process, perhaps an assessment form for high risk of falls, and then walk away. If the data reveal that falls have not decreased once the new form has been implemented, then the intervention did not provide either the patient or the institution with any suffering decreases, everyone benefits—the patient and the organization. When patients benefit and don't die unnecessarily and they have fewer complications, that's value. Also, documenting compliance with this evidence-based measure is part of the CMS initiative to reward hospitals financially.

Linking process and outcome measures is also useful for developing an approach to prevention. If data analysis reveals that although the physician writes an order for aspirin, it is not filled or delivered, a problem with the process is identified. Once a problem is recognized, it behooves leaders to discover the cause of the gap in safety and to hold someone accountable. Often there are so many caregivers involved with a single patient that no one knows who is responsible for what. The primary physician has to maintain responsibility and assign someone the task of administering the aspirin in a timely way to the correct patient. That aspirin delivery also has to be properly documented—not simply to comply with CMS standards but also to maintain a record of proper care in the medical chart to reduce errors and improve communication. The physician should assign the task of documentation as well. If a physician writes an order or orders aspirin over the phone and then relinquishes responsibility, that is a failure in the process. If the physician accepts accountability for the delivery of aspirin and develops a process and procedure in which expectations of various staff members are clear, everyone benefits—that is value.

value. Staff education based on data increases the value of the measure. When staff realize that falls are ongoing and affecting a large patient population (the elderly), and that the organization's insurance rates are rising due to malpractice claims, they also realize the clinical and organizational benefit of ensuring appropriate care.

There may be numerous causes of patient falls and therefore analysis is necessary to reveal the underlying reasons before the organization can formulate corrective action. Perhaps a caregiver is slow in responding to the patient's call bell, and the patient attempts to ambulate without assistance. Perhaps the patient has medication, such as a diuretic, that increases urination, and the patient requires frequent visits to the toilet but is reluctant to call staff and tries to get up alone. Perhaps the patient is taking medication that affects balance or increases disorientation. Or perhaps there is some obstruction or poor lighting in the environment of the patient's room or bathroom. Patients might fall for any or all of these reasons or for other reasons. Once the cause of the falls is understood, processes can be put in place to prevent them.

ASKING QUESTIONS VIA DATA

Before a health care organization invests in data collection efforts, it is crucial to know what is being examined, what question is being asked, what assumption is being tested, and why. In other words, for a collection effort to be meaningful, you need to know why you are collecting the data and how you hope to use the information revealed by the data.

Imagine that the members of a medical board are discussing postoperative bleeding and its consequences. Clinical leaders would like to understand this negative phenomenon, which is dangerous for the patients and costly to the organization. Why are patients bleeding after surgical procedures? Is the bleeding related to a particular population or a particular disease process? Is it from lack of technical competence? Is it possibly happening because the patients were not properly assessed as viable candidates for surgery? Or is it happening because blood-thinning medication was not stopped before surgery?

There are many potential reasons, and each has an impact on how information is collected. The question being asked defines the type of data being gathered and the methodology used. An intelligent place to begin to examine the problem is by interviewing clinicians and, along with quality professionals, examining the medical records of patients who suffered postoperative bleeding. A root cause analysis of each bleeding episode should be undertaken in order to define the various factors involved in the problem.

Root Cause Analysis

A root cause analysis (RCA) is a quality management tool that dissects a situation into its components in order to discover weaknesses and defects in a process. Through a careful analysis of the event, variables can be identified that may have contributed to a poor outcome. These variables may involve equipment, human resources, documentation, communication, technology, policies and procedures, or other relevant categories.

Root cause analysis reveals where gaps in care exist and where mistakes are made. Usually multiple factors are involved in any adverse event. Rarely can a single cause be pinpointed as the culprit. Quality management uses the metaphor of Swiss cheese to explain how processes become vulnerable. Mistakes (holes in the process) occur here and there, some larger and more significant than others. Eventually several holes line up and the patient falls through; once the patient is harmed, people take notice. When holes are identified before they can line up and great harm is done, the process can be repaired.

The variables in the process or procedure being analyzed can be represented graphically in a fishbone diagram (see Figure 2.2), also called an Ishikawa diagram (after its creator, Kaoru Ishikawa). By drawing a fishbone diagram for a poor outcome, analysts can first categorize the larger "bones"—the primary causes of the problem—and then drill down to the smaller "bones" for each primary cause.

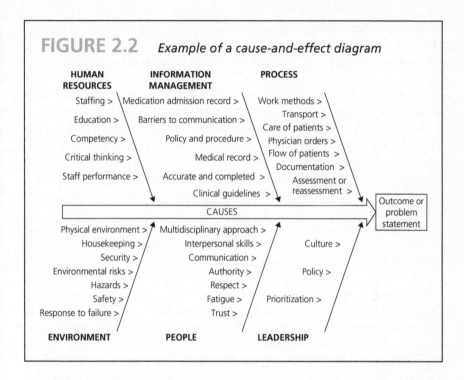

FIGURE 2.2   *Example of a cause-and-effect diagram*

In the past each area found by a root cause analysis to be involved in a poor outcome would have been assigned a corrective action. However, some organizations then realized that those corrective actions were not sustained. Now, rather than introduce a series of changes in practice, these organizations "weigh" the bones and through consensus with the analytical team, they ascertain which areas are most relevant to producing the outcome. Thus the initial fishbone becomes a kind of filter to identify the most critical areas that require improvements. Once those areas are defined, another fishbone, drilling down in those areas, is developed and becomes the focus of the corrective action.

Once corrections are developed and implemented, data reports should be generated to track their effectiveness, with periodic reports given to relevant groups. Ongoing data collection will reveal which changes have been integrated into the process of care and which have not. If there has been little change after the intervention, go back to the drawing board. You need to try another intervention, collect data on its effectiveness, and report your findings.

Data Analysis Leads to Improvements

Once the cause of an error is identified, regulations require that the health care organization take corrective actions—steps to improve. That's the point, after all, to improve by reducing faulty processes and increasing patient safety.

By aggregating information on several patients, leaders may be able to formulate an assumption to investigate. For example, if root cause analysis points to the preparation of the surgical site as a factor in the negative complication of infection, then information about surgical site and postoperative complications would be collected and tracked. A medical record review might reveal the frequency of the problem and what patient population or medical condition is most vulnerable to the procedure. Perhaps the postoperative care is inadequate because of inadequate staffing or staff who are not appropriately educated and trained. Some surgeries require specialists in that surgery to monitor the patient's postsurgical progress. The point here is that data collection should be done for a reason, and with an idea, hypothesis, or concern as motivation.

Data collectors require training, especially when clinical or technical data are being collected. If a medical chart is being reviewed for information, training should be conducted by clinicians to alert data collectors to the appropriate variables. Reading and interpreting a medical record for information may require analysis of qualitative notes. For example, should the preoperative assessment be the target of inquiry (perhaps blood-thinning medication should have been stopped before surgery), or should the postoperative medication regimen be examined, or should the data collector be on the lookout for any special comorbidities that might have had an impact on the adverse result? You cannot just plow into a database (the medical record is a database) assuming that relevant information will jump off the page. Quality management staff and clinicians can develop training and educational programs to assist data collection efforts.

The goal of the analysis is to discover why an adverse event occurred and to put in place procedures to minimize the risk. Once attention is focused on the problem, clinical staff are more responsive to warning signs and cues that suggest a potential complication. Analysis avoids the traditional blame approach to poor outcomes; blame usually results in defensive arguments. Often I hear clinicians suggest that a poor outcome was an artifact of a clerical error, that the coding of the diagnosis was inaccurate, or that their patients as a group are very old (eighty-five or more) and come from nursing homes where they receive only palliative care and therefore the clinicians are not responsible for the results or outcomes.

Amount of Data to Collect

Many people do not know how much data should be collected and over how long a time. Again, the amount of data needed depends on the question or problem being examined. Let's say you want to know how many obstetrical patients suffer bleeding after a cesarean section (C-section). You can look back at one year's worth of charts, identify the patients who had a bleeding episode, and then develop an audit tool with the obstetricians to distinguish clinical factors such as underlying diseases or conditions. The charts of those patients with clinical problems should be further analyzed by peer review.

You want to know whether the bleeding episodes can be correlated with any other factor, such as age, physiology, type of delivery, predelivery assessment, medication, or experience of the physician. If the problem occurs primarily at night, when the resident house staff are on duty, does the lack of experience in recognizing the warning signs of trouble explain the data? If the peer review finds that this is the case, educational programs or changes in policies and procedures should be instituted.

Sample Size

Another factor to consider when collecting data is sample size—how many patients do you need to consider to come to a valid conclusion about a question or hypothesis? Often it is impractical to collect data on an entire population; therefore data are collected on a subset that represents the larger population. From the results of the sample, the researcher makes inferences about the larger population. A general rule of thumb is to sample 10 percent of the total population if it is large or 100 percent if the population under review has fewer than fifty members. Medical records should be selected randomly. (Textbooks on statistics provide information about random selection.)

Data Validity

I have found that when I present physicians with data about processes and results and those data reveal gaps in care or unsafe practices or poor results, the physicians are frequently skeptical about the accuracy of the data. Administrative data that are used for billing reveal only the broadest factors: who, how long, what for, and with what result. Physicians correctly suspect that these data do not reflect the complexity of care. Therefore to convince physicians to change their practice, it is crucial to ensure that the data not only are accurate and valid but are also from an appropriate source, such as the medical record.

For data to be meaningful to physicians, they should be risk adjusted. Risk adjustment is a statistical process that ensures that patients are appropriately classified together so that comparisons are valid. The data are adjusted for variation, especially in those characteristics that affect outcome. Data on cardiac mortality, for example, are risk adjusted for comorbidities (such as heart failure, pneumonia, hypertension, diabetes), age, or other factors that might contribute to an explanation of case severity. In order to explain variations from established benchmarks, it is necessary to compare patients at similar severity levels.

PRESENTING RESULTS

Working with information technology (IT) and quality management personnel, researchers can construct databases with appropriate statistical tools. Generally data are collected over a number of months, to avoid reporting chance occurrences or idiosyncratic results. Tables are useful in defining relationships among variables. To ascertain whether or not variables are matched in a cause and effect relationship, analysts should do a regression analysis if such an analysis is appropriate for answering a question. Again, IT staff are trained to help health care workers establish and interpret reliable data.

Once the data are collected and interpreted, the results of the analysis should be presented to the appropriate caregivers and administrators. Information lying in a drawer or sitting in a computer file does no one any good.

Data should be displayed in such a way that others can visualize the information. Graphs, tables, charts, and bulleted lists are usually effective ways to communicate information and educate an audience about how to use data for improvements.

It is helpful to use appropriate formats to display different kinds of information. There are numerous ways in addition to fishbone diagrams and tables of measures to present quality data effectively. One method is the run chart, a continuous graph that exposes trends over time. Figure 2.3, for example, shows a run chart that tracks the volume of pneumonia cases for one hospital over time. The chart reveals that the hospital had the greatest number of pneumonia patients in January. With this information, leaders may want to increase staff or provide more services during anticipated high patient population periods.

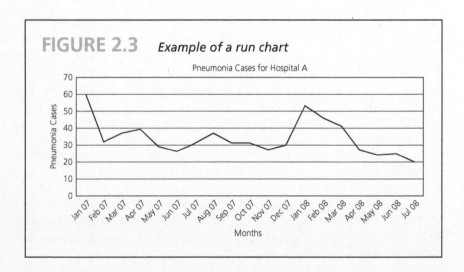

FIGURE 2.3 *Example of a run chart*

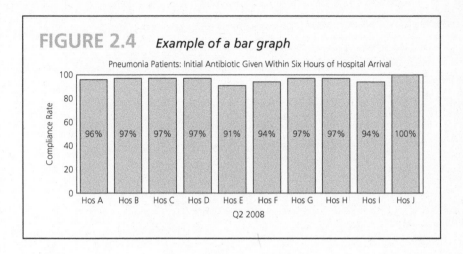

FIGURE 2.4 *Example of a bar graph*

Pneumonia Patients: Initial Antibiotic Given Within Six Hours of Hospital Arrival

Another way to display data is a bar graph, which uses bars of varying height or width to compare different categories. The graph in Figure 2.4, for example, compares the quarterly compliance rate of ten hospitals in a health system on the measure of antibiotic administration within six hours of arrival for pneumonia patients. The goal for compliance is 100 percent, a goal achieved by Hospital J. Hospital E shows the lowest compliance rate for the quarter. Leaders can see at a glance which hospitals are more successful than others. They may suggest that Hospital J communicate its best practices to Hospital E in order to make improvements.

Pie charts can reveal at a glance how various factors relate to each other on a measure. Figure 2.5, for example, displays information about the ethnicity of stroke patients. A pie chart helps stakeholders visualize relative percentages among an entire patient population. This chart reveals that most stroke patients were white and that the next largest category was African American. Leaders might use this information to introduce educational efforts in the appropriate community venues.

Control charts are used to monitor the stability of a process. The chart displaying the number of days that patients in the ICU are on central lines for infection in Figure 2.6, for instance, shows the variations from the mean over time and which processes are in control. When processes are seen to be outside either the upper control limit (UCL) or lower control limit (LCL), an investigation of the reasons can be conducted.

To whom should data be reported? In order to close the loop, results should be reported to organizational staff and decision makers and also to those invested in asking questions about care. Hospitals are charged by the Joint Commission to maintain and monitor quality of care and patient safety through *tracer methodology* and survey readiness.

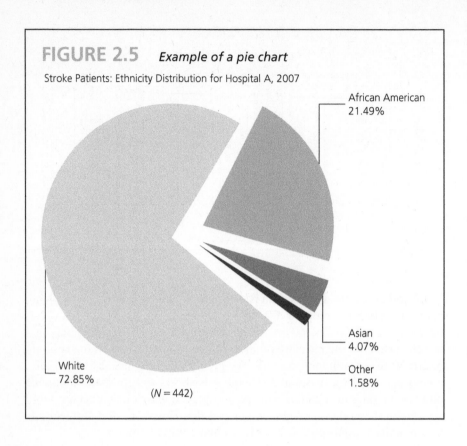

FIGURE 2.5 *Example of a pie chart*

Stroke Patients: Ethnicity Distribution for Hospital A, 2007

African American
21.49%

White
72.85%

Asian
4.07%

Other
1.58%

(*N* = 442)

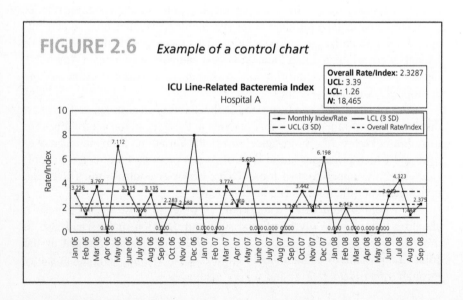

FIGURE 2.6 *Example of a control chart*

Overall Rate/Index: 2.3287
UCL: 3.39
LCL: 1.26
N: 18,465

ICU Line-Related Bacteremia Index
Hospital A

Monthly Index/Rate — LCL (3 SD)
— — UCL (3 SD) — — — Overall Rate/Index

TRACER METHODOLOGY Tracer methodology evaluates an organization's compliance with standards by focusing on the specifics of a patient's care as he or she moves through the care continuum from the ED or routine admission through the course of treatment to discharge. Tracers use data to examine the care of a varied selection of patients—such as high-risk patients, patients who come to the ED with multiple diagnoses, and patients who come from nursing homes with an acute situation—to ensure that the care delivered is appropriate. Joint Commission surveyors question staff and clinicians about each selected patient's specific care processes. The goal is to assess compliance with standards so that all patients are ensured safe care. This methodology also helps clinicians to focus on the patient, the process of care, and the outcome of treatment, and it helps organizations to focus on the continuum of care and the relationships among the different units that patients experience during an episode of hospitalization.

EFFECTIVE COMMUNICATION IMPROVES PATIENT SAFETY

The quality committee of the board of trustees is responsible for maintaining oversight of care. Information can and should be reported to the quality committee. Many organizations also have performance improvement (PI) committees. These committees are multidisciplinary and can be an effective way to carry information throughout the organization. Not only physicians and nurses, quality staff, and administrators but also respiratory specialists, nutritionists, social workers, risk managers, dieticians, engineers, and so on can be present at PI committee meetings. Once information is reported, they should take it back to their unit or department or service and communicate it to their staff. The idea is to get the word out there.

Figure 2.7 illustrates how information can travel from an individual site's quality management department to a systemwide quality management meeting to performance improvement committees and to the board of trustees. The intent of this committee structure is to ensure that the quality process is maintained, that accountability is built in to sustain change, and that improvements can be monitored over time. The board should receive hospital services data monthly and these data should be analyzed and explained. Ongoing reports will reinforce lines of communication that help to create a culture of quality and safety. These reports should be generated by the quality management department. The focus of each report can be on outcomes (such as mortality) and on results of peer reviews resulting from indications that the standard of care has not been met.

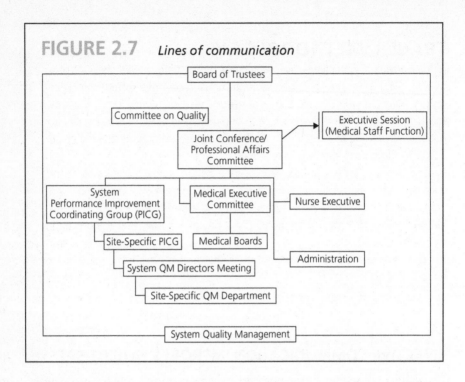

FIGURE 2.7 *Lines of communication*

For example, needlestick (or sharps) injuries are a safety concern for employees. Their health can be jeopardized, and work days can be lost. If leadership prioritizes sharps safety and asks quality management personnel to collect and track data about these injuries, having an established communication structure will formalize the transfer of this information from the bedside, where the injury occurs, to the middle managers and through various committees to the medical board and board of trustees. With this information, leaders can evaluate improvement efforts. Did the number of injuries go up or down? If the changes made are not resulting in improvements, why not? By creating a communication structure for quality information to travel throughout the organization, the organization makes everyone involved a part of the improvement efforts.

Having a report back process is also essential. Often information and good ideas get stalled at meetings, with the frontline staff remaining unaware of proposed changes in procedures. This is one of the major obstacles to creating a culture of quality and safety. Managers should take the responsibility for keeping their staff informed, and the medical board should clearly define who is accountable for informing people about and implementing improvements and changes for various services and departments. And the improvement effort should not stop there. The medical board should require regular updates about the success of improvements. Data that are reported back to the PI committees will help to close the loop.

SUMMARY

Improvements to patient safety

- Rely on aggregated, objective data to drive clinical decisions
- Involve multidisciplinary teams that can recommend and implement changed practices
- Reflect improved organizational efficiency
- Result from understanding and analyzing gaps in patient safety
- Require effective and ongoing communication through appropriate performance improvement reports

KEY TERMS

benchmark
hospital culture
quality indicator

root cause analysis
tracer methodology

THINGS TO THINK ABOUT

If you were the CFO of a community hospital, what types of data would you collect and analyze to ensure that resources were being spent effectively and efficiently?

1. What measures would you use?
2. Once data have been analyzed, how would you communicate the resulting information, and to whom?
3. What steps would you take to ensure more efficient processes in the delivery of care?

CHAPTER

3

FOCUS ON THE PATIENT

LEARNING OBJECTIVES

- Describe the role of communication in a patient-focused environment of care, with the treatment plan as a unit of analysis
- Discuss barriers to effective communication and strategies to overcome them
- Describe the value of using clinical guidelines and pathways to promote a patient-focused environment
- Explain the importance of patient education in promoting good outcomes
- Explain the importance of documenting near misses to improve patient safety

Health care in this country is moving from a treatment- or task-focused approach to a patient-focused one. Such an approach involves bringing the patient and family into the treatment loop, with tools, explanations, improved communication, and information for intelligent decision making. For this approach to succeed, everyone involved in patient care, from the physician and nurse to the ancillary staff, has to be committed to and educated about patient-focused care. Administrators must also be committed and educated because this approach is more time consuming for caregivers and may be perceived as not as efficient as more traditional, task-oriented care.

In fact patient-focused care is more efficient and cost effective. As I will explain in this chapter, patient-focused care saves money, uses fewer expensive resources, improves public relations and patient satisfaction, and most important, improves patient care. Moving from a focus on the treatment or task to a focus on the patient encourages caregivers to assess the patient's response to treatment. In a patient-focused environment the patient's environment and health status are considered on an ongoing basis.

For example, when nurses are administering medication, their traditional focus is on completing the task within a specified period of time. In this approach the nurse moves from patient to patient, giving out medication, and the interaction between the nurse and the patient is minimal; the nurse is concerned with correct patient identification, correct drug identification, and correct administration. These are indeed important tasks, and if performed poorly they may result in errors. The wrong patient might get the medication, the patient might get the wrong medication, the medication might be delivered in the wrong way (perhaps through an IV rather than orally), or the dosage might be wrong. Managing these tasks requires the nurse to focus on the delivery of the medication.

In a patient-focused environment the patient is central, with communication going both ways. The nurse assesses the patient's condition and health status prior to the administration of the medication and checks the patient's status after the medication is administered to ensure that the intervention has had the desired effect. Naturally, this approach may take more time. However, it reduces the potential for errors, misadministrations, and adverse drug reactions—all these events are costly in terms of time and resources to manage and correct.

In a patient-focused environment the caregiver addresses issues beyond the medical that might also have an impact on the well-being of the patient. For example, chronic diseases, such as congestive heart failure (CHF), require tremendous health care resources, so many hospitals and health care organizations are attempting to improve care and efficiency in these cases by focusing on the patient rather than the disease process. It may be important to understand the patient's emotional state, which might make a difference in terms of compliance with treatment, and the patient's living situation, which might also make a difference. If the caregiver assesses the health literacy of the patient, that information might be used to guide education about disease management and improve how well the patient manages. Patient-focused care requires more time from the caregiver than treatment-focused care does. But the results may be better and more efficient. The goal is to avoid readmission through helping the patient understand the importance of medication, exercise, nutrition, and medical follow-up in the treatment and management of his or her CHF.

Leaders need to accept and approve the resources for this model of care. It may require more staff. The pay-for-performance measures gathered nationally by the Centers for Medicare and Medicaid Services (CMS) indicate that patients who are discharged with CHF do not get adequate and effective information. Reimbursement for health care is refocusing payment on processes of care to improve the health care status of patients with chronic diseases. Ironically, because money is involved, administrative leaders are putting pressure on clinicians to change, for example, their attitude toward discharge. CEOs are applying extra pressure on middle managers and compensating them with financial incentives to ensure compliance with the process measure established by CMS. The pay-for-performance measures, when applied appropriately, encourage the multidisciplinary team to address patient needs beyond the hospital and into the community and to define patients' long-term needs.

Patients are no longer passive recipients of often unintelligible information. I have even seen patients researching medical information on the Internet as they lie in a hospital bed. Patients expect to be involved in their care. Advocacy groups and regulatory agencies have fostered an awareness of patients' role in medical care that has led to the movement toward transparency, with the goal of providing clear information, explicit treatment plans, and complete documentation detailing safe and appropriate care.

EFFECTIVE COMMUNICATION AND PATIENT-FOCUSED CARE

Underlying the patient-focused movement and the push toward transparency is effective communication. It seems obvious that communication about patient care should be effective, but patients have been expressing their sense of isolation and their confusion and lack of understanding about their illnesses, their treatments, and their discharge instructions for a very long time.

In a patient-focused environment the caregiving team is focused not only on the immediate problem but also on managing the patient throughout the continuum of care—not an easy or simple task. Often this responsibility is assigned to a nurse (whose title is, for example, care coordinator) and his or her role is to communicate with the different physicians on the team. Effective communication can streamline treatment and increase value through developing processes for highly coordinated, focused, and efficient care. Social workers play a major role in explaining the emotional and social condition of the patient. The team approach also leads to early discharge and a short and appropriate length of stay (LOS) that results in saving money.

All the caregiving team members meet daily to do rounds on each patient, with the assigned nurse coordinating information. The communication is about the patient, about the effectiveness of treatment, and about ensuring that the patient is receiving the appropriate level of care. Coordinating care among the all the doctors, nurses, social workers, nutritionists, respiratory therapists, and so on requires a commitment of time but in most cases results in reduced readmission rates.

Poor communication is almost always a factor in medical errors and can be identified through root cause analysis. Problems can occur due to a lack of documentation, which has a negative impact in that consultations are not timely, assessments or reassessments of the patient's condition are not adequately performed, and monitoring of the effectiveness of treatment is not timely. Documentation is essential to the delivery of quality care. It is not just paper! Documentation articulates information about the patient that cannot be found anywhere else and is necessary for the coordination of care among various caregivers.

Often verbal communication is not documented in the medical record, which also results in misinformation and failures of communication. Staff changes and handoffs are vulnerable to communication failures because the information does not travel with the patient as she or he moves through the continuum, or it does not move from staff to staff at shift changes. Even when the medical record is appropriately documented, communication failures can occur through a failure to read through it.

Figure 3.1 displays how information must be moved across multiple facilities and various cycles in an episode of hospitalization. From the physician's office through admission and treatment to discharge and home care posthospitalization, knowledge must be shared. Failures in information transfer are among the best-known risks to patient safety associated with moving patients along the continuum of care. What this means is that as a patient moves from the physician's office to the hospital inpatient unit, and perhaps to surgery, postsurgical care, step-down units, and rehabilitation or home care, safety has to be preserved and consistent throughout. Documentation about treatment has to be complete and timely at each stage along the continuum for caregivers to be properly informed.

As the population ages, patients are entering hospitals with multiple and complex physical conditions that require multiple interventions controlled by numerous caregivers. Often unanticipated complications occur, such as falls

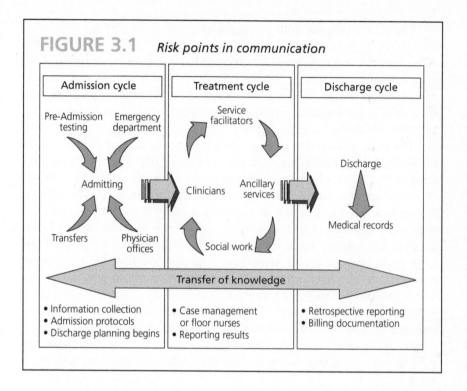

FIGURE 3.1 *Risk points in communication*

(to which the elderly are particularly susceptible), which can require surgery (involving more and different caregivers) or lead to blood clots or other problems. As patients move along the continuum of care, there may be failures of communication that also cause inefficiencies or poor outcomes. Clinicians can no longer be out of the loop of utilization management (traditionally separated from clinical care) or discharge planning. Patients receive better quality care and the organization can be more cost effective when all the individuals involved work together.

In order to facilitate effective communication, organizations should explicitly define and design processes that formalize communication, whether this involves standardizing documentation in the medical record, ensuring that entries are timely, or developing techniques to ensure that oral or written information is effectively transferred among different caregivers. Leaders must support these explicit efforts to standardize and improve communication or staff will not buy into new processes. Finally, the effectiveness of communication should be evaluated via data and reported throughout the organization. Standardized tools and a team approach should be adopted as a normal routine of care.

One of the preconditions to establishing any change in the delivery of care is having the explicit support of administrative and clinical leadership. Administrative support should be reflected in the budget, with financial and other resources allocated to promote a focus on quality and safety. Clinicians have to be encouraged to bring the patient into the treatment plan, allowing the patient to ask questions, to proactively engage in decisions about care, and to communicate with care providers.

The goal of focusing clinical attention on the patient is to create an environment that encourages communication for improved outcomes. The hope is that by involving patients there may be fewer adverse events and increased organizational efficiency. Some of the burden falls on the patients themselves. Patients can and should remind caregivers about any allergies they have; patients should be able to report their medications, including dosages. Patients are asked for identification throughout their hospital stay in order to prevent events associated with misidentification. Patients are required to explicitly verify the site of surgery with the surgical team in an attempt to avoid wrong-site surgeries. Without active patient participation, it is possible for busy caregivers to make mistakes, especially during shift transfers or when patients move along the continuum of care. With fewer errors and adverse events, organizational processes move more smoothly than they do when there are problems that disrupt the efficient delivery of services.

Errors create crises. Normal care activities have to stop in order for staff to manage the crisis. The normal process of care is disrupted, and the additional work uses clinician time and hospital resources. Often patients need to be transferred to another level of care, such as the intensive care unit (ICU), because of new problems associated with an error. Time-consuming reports have to be filed with accreditation authorities or the department of health; root cause analyses are required to understand the gaps in care and develop corrective actions. Patients and families must be notified of the error.

Focusing attention on the whole patient rather than on the clinical task reduces errors and promotes improved organizational efficiency, especially when care management is aggregated by disease. Caregivers can then plan for tests and laboratory work by patient populations, helping to avoid bottlenecks, and the pharmacy can order medications on the basis of numbers, saving the organization money. Patients can also be educated about the value of different levels of care and the role of informed consent in explaining potential complications and risks. When the patients make decisions based on information, there are better results.

It takes years to move from a traditional paradigm of the delivery of care to a patient-focused environment. It is easy to make a quick fix, change a process, and even put it into effect. What is more difficult is sustaining the change so that new processes become a routine part of the hospital culture.

HANDOFF INFORMATION TRANSFER

According to the Joint Commission's sentinel event database, the primary cause of adverse events, as shown through root cause analyses, is poor communication. A primary objective of the new Joint Commission recommendation for standardizing communication during a patient "handoff" is to transfer accurate and timely information about the patient's condition and treatment. Handoff communication is a real-time process of transferring information from one caregiver to another to ensure continuity and safety of care. Common opportunities for handoffs are shift changes (when nurses who are going off duty pass information along to the next shift), and the movement of patients along the continuum of care (for example, from the emergency department [ED] to a medical unit or from a medical unit to a nursing or long-term care facility).

Another place where information transfer is critical is among the medical or clinical staff when a physician who is used to working in isolation has to provide timely and complete information to another specialist. Also, when a patient is seeing multiple specialists, someone has to be in charge, and that means also in charge of effective communication. Yet other opportunities for handoffs occur between a patient's nurse and the physician and between the nurse and ancillary personnel, where accuracy, completeness, and timeliness are again crucial to maintaining patient safety.

SBAR

The SBAR technique is designed to focus attention on effective and efficient communication. It is useful for standardizing communication, especially during those vulnerable spots of information transfer and handoffs. Integrated into this standardized approach is the opportunity to ask questions. Obviously, if one is just reading a hastily scribbled note in a medical record, there is no such opportunity.

SBAR is an acronym that stands for *s*ituation, *b*ackground, *a*ssessment, and *r*ecommendations. Although it seems obvious that communicating about a patient's condition might involve information about each of these concepts, having a handy mnemonic and standardizing its application across the entire hospital helps to clearly define communication expectations. Especially useful in today's complex medical environment with complex patients, SBAR is intended to simplify as well as standardize communication. With such a defined and proscribed framework, communication is replicable between caregivers. The goal of this technique is not only to control the effectiveness and content of communication but also, by doing so, to avoid risks to patients.

The hope is to use standardization to maximize the transmission of critical information. Communicating the *situation* involves stating the patient's name, age, and unit; the time of admission; and the assessment. It also involves defining the problem one is communicating about—diagnosis, treatment options, or placement. Communicating the *background* involves supplying information about the relevant medical history; previous hospitalizations, if any; medications and the reasons for them; and what has occurred from admission to the moment of communication. Communicating the *assessment* involves supplying the results of the history and physical and the vital signs, imaging studies, laboratory values, and so on, as well as any other pertinent information acquired since admission. Also, it is important to describe any changes that have occurred since the previous encounter or assessment. Communicating the *recommendations* means stating any need for consultations, a time frame for further evaluations, a timetable for clinical and medical management, and discharge recommendations (where? when?). The intent of the SBAR technique is to offer the receiving caregiver a complete and timely report on the status of the patient.

BARRIERS TO EFFECTIVE COMMUNICATION

Obviously, caregivers require information. This is so obvious that one might ask why a regulatory agency needs to mandate effective communication. Why is the communication of information during a handoff a high-risk activity? What impedes effective communication among caregivers? There may be many answers to these questions: constraints of time, as caregivers are often managing many patients at once; gauging the correct amount of information to transfer, neither too much nor too little; documenting appropriately in the medical record so that caregivers have information about treatments and interventions and their effectiveness for the patient.

Also, some simple human factors impede communication: people forget, are distracted, have different levels of communication ability and language skill (for example, they may have illegible handwriting or use inappropriate abbreviations), and may have priorities relating to their specialization, making one type of information more salient to them than another. Moreover, health care organizations often have implicit hierarchies of power, and subordinates may not feel comfortable communicating with someone higher up on the chain.

Cultural barriers also affect communication. Physicians are trained to trust themselves and to make their own decisions based on their experience and training. They are not trained to be team members or particularly effective communicators. They are also used to being the captain of the ship, with their orders going unquestioned by staff. It is difficult to change such entrenched attitudes. Within the hierarchy of the hospital staff are many opportunities for failures of communication. The attending physician's orders

EXAMPLE: MISHANDLED PATHOLOGY SAMPLE

One example of a poor patient outcome resulting from a failure of communication involved a patient who had had a double mastectomy. A nurse was expected to transport the tissue specimens collected during surgery to a refrigerator for storage until they could be collected by pathology for analysis. When the nurse went to place the specimens in the refrigerator, a physician was standing in front of it, blocking access. The nurse was new to the organization and was shy. She was uncomfortable with asking the physician to move and she put the specimens on the desk, intending to wait and then refrigerate them after the physician had left.

However, as often happens, an emergency occurred and the nurse was urgently called to the operating room. She forgot all about the specimens. By the time someone noticed the specimens on the desk, it was too late for micropathology to be performed. Due to social and culture factors, rather than medical ones, the patient's outcome and safety were affected.

EXAMPLE: INCORRECT DRUG DOSAGE

In an effort to reduce medication errors, a hospital developed policies to promote accurate communication among caregivers. Multiple redundancies were instituted in order to establish fail-safe processes. One policy dictated that the surgeon is expected to communicate to the anesthesiologist about medication; the anesthesiologist is expected to concur, if appropriate, that the medication order is correct and to communicate that order to the nurse, who then is expected to repeat and validate the order. The reason for this policy is to reduce errors by having multiple safeguards, with several clinicians confirming the order.

In one incident, however, the surgeon requested the medication directly from the nurse, leaving the anesthesiologist out of the loop. The nurse did not confirm the order with the anesthesiologist either. The result of not following procedure was that the surgeon injected the wrong concentration of medication into the patient, causing cardiac arrest.

Miscommunications such as this are not uncommon. Clinicians are rushed, think they know what they are doing, are impatient with protocols that require repetition and multiple approvals, and arrogantly do what they do. Often such shortcuts result in patient harm.

may not be clear, the resident may not question an unclear order, or the nurse may not feel comfortable asking the physician for something.

STRATEGIES TO REDUCE BARRIERS

The first requirement in making change is a willingness to change. Change is hard in most circumstances, and in the established health care environment, it is especially difficult. Too many individual agendas, too many experts working in silos, a very powerful and long-established hierarchy, and a separation of administrative and clinical oversight—all these factors make change exceedingly difficult. In addition to a willingness to entertain new ideas and to change established practices, a leadership commitment is required. Without it any change is doomed to be short lived. Leaders have to be clear and committed about wanting something to change and to improve, and they must want to see the results of the change on an ongoing basis.

Once there is a willingness to entertain change, some tools and techniques can help bring it about. First and foremost is proof, in the form of data, that something is wrong. Infection rates that are higher than average; mortality rates that are higher; high rates of patient falls, staff turnover, LOS—all indicate problems and inefficient processes. Once it is decided that change is called for, establishing multidisciplinary teams to determine specific improvements encourages buy-in from staff, much more so than change dictated from one person. The more staff who are involved in an improvement effort, and the more representatives from the departments, services, and disciplines that might be affected by the change who are involved, the more likely it is that multiple agendas will be addressed.

Education is crucial to help people interpret data as useful information, to promote communication around an issue, and to establish a climate of collaboration and trust. Led by organization leaders, efforts should be made to change from a mainly reactive model of care to a mainly proactive one. In the reactive model caregivers are busy responding to emergencies, and they spend most days dealing with crises, putting out fires as they occur. In other words, they react to what is happening around them. A proactive model is different. It anticipates potential areas of risk to patients and, before a crisis develops, puts policies and procedures in place to try to avoid these problems or prevent them from ever happening.

A proactive analysis uses a technique called failure mode and effects analysis (FMEA), which involves staff in analyzing potential areas for improvement. In the proactive model of care, the end goal is quality and best practices; in the reactive model, which uses tools such as root cause analysis (RCA), the goal is to understand problems that have already occurred in order to foster improvement. Both types of analysis are useful for improving care. Table 3.1 shows what both types share and how they differ.

TABLE 3.1 Methodology for error analysis

RCA	FMEA
Both are nonstatistical methods of analysis	
Both have a goal of reducing patient harm	
Both identify conditions that lead to harm	
Both are interdisciplinary team activities	
Reactive	Proactive
Focuses on event	Focuses on entire process
Hindsight bias	Unbiased
Fear; resistance	Openness
Asks "Why?"	Asks "What?"

Another technique to improve care through establishing methods for improved communication has been formalized by the Institute for Healthcare Improvement (IHI). It involves forming rapid response teams (RRTs) trained to cope with emergencies quickly and in a standardized way. This model, based on the Code Blue approach used for heart attacks, calls a multidisciplinary team to the patient's bedside during an emergency or crisis. Staff report great satisfaction with RRTs because of their timely and efficient response to a call for help.

CARE AND COMMUNICATION GUIDELINES

Another effective tool used to improve communication and coordinate activities among multiple caregivers is the clinical pathway. Clinical pathways are disease-specific plans of care developed by clinician specialists. They are based on nationally recognized clinical guidelines for appropriate care for various diseases, and they incorporate evidence-based medicine, which means that they include proven algorithms for care based on the most comprehensive, up-to-date research and clinical expertise. Their intent is to improve patient outcomes through improving communication among caregivers and eliminating the silos of disparate disciplines in order to reduce variation in the way care is delivered, to maintain continuity of care throughout an episode of hospitalization, to maximize the efficient use of resources, and finally to locate gaps in the delivery of care that can then be reduced. For all these reasons clinical pathways and other kinds of guidelines are supported by health care agencies and organizations.

In outlining evidence-based care and the appropriate time frame for that care, pathways define what should be done, in what order, and by whom. Interventions and expected outcomes are listed daily on each patient's pathway, which leads to organizational efficiency. Nurses and other health care clinicians know what has been done, with what effect, and what's next in the treatment plan. Best of all, this information is in one place—on the pathway—and not scattered in notes throughout the patient's chart.

A great benefit of using a clinical pathway is that during shift changes, where studies show communication gaps are frequent and patients are vulnerable to errors, the oncoming shift can see at a glance the daily progress and health status of the patient. Other advantages of putting patients on pathways are increased caregiver collaboration and improved organizational efficiency as a result of planning prospectively for care. Also, accountability is better defined and strengthened because there is a clear link between assessment and interventions with outcomes.

Clinical pathways focus caregivers' attention on measures. For example, evidence indicates that patients who are diagnosed with pneumonia should move from intravenous (IV) to oral antibiotics on day 3 of treatment (see Figure 3.2). They should also have an established discharge plan. These and other measures are outlined on the pathway, reminding caregivers about them and also providing space for documentation of compliance. Health care administrators encourage compliance with these measures because the organization gets paid for complying with recommended measures. Pathways also remind physicians about the importance of managing the subacute phase of hospitalization.

PATIENT EDUCATION

Hospitals are also preparing pamphlets and informational videos to educate patients about their hospitalization. For example, many hospitals use special assessment tools to identify patients at high risk for falling. Staff are assigned to high-risk patients to reduce falls. But another and often overlooked component to reducing the risk of falls is to educate patients themselves about the risk and the potential complications of falling, which can be life threatening if appropriate care is not maintained.

FIGURE 3.2 *Pneumonia guideline, clinical version*

		PNEUMONIA GUIDELINE Clinical Version	
		INTERVENTIONS	OUTCOMES
ASSESSMENT	TESTS		Patient's white blood cell count is returning to normal
	MONITORS AND TEAM PROCESS	Daily assessment/reassessment	Patient's temperature is below 38.3°C
		Vital signs every: _____	Patient can take oral medications
		Aspiration precautions	Patient's respiratory rate is at or below 24
		Assess skin	Patient's systolic BP is above 90 and below 160
		Intake and output	Patient's pulse is below 100
			Patient's mental status is at baseline
PLAN	TREATMENTS	Deep breathe and cough/use of incentive spirometry	
		Oxygen as ordered: _____	
		IV: _____	
		Encourage fluids (if not contraindicated)	
		DVT prophylaxis	
		Pulse oximetry every: _____ hours	
	MEDICATIONS	Consider switch from IV antibiotics to oral antibiotics if appropriate	Patient/Significant Other verbalize an understanding of the medication regimen
		Antibiotics	
		Inhalation therapy as ordered	
		Pain management	
	DIET	As orde [INTERVENTION — Consider switch from IV antibiotics to oral antibiotics if appropriate] _____	Patie [OUTCOME — Patient or significant other verbalizes an understanding of the medication regimen]
	ACTIVITY	As orde _____	Patie perio ... rest
	TEACHING	Review medications and smoking cessation/effects of second hand smoke	
	DISCHARGE PLANNING	Discharge plan established	Patient or significant Other agrees with the discharge plan
		Determine if home oxygen is indicated	

Information is made available to patients in an attempt to increase their knowledge about medical care and to involve them in their care. For example, New York State provides cardiac surgery patients with booklets that explain the surgery, the procedures involved, what to expect, and what the mortality rates are at different health care institutions. The American Medical Association (AMA) has published guidelines to educate people to recognize symptoms of a stroke or heart attack. It also has guidelines on preventing infections, including making sure that caregivers wash their hands before patient contact.

Such booklets offer information that helps patients make choices about where to go for their medical care. By offering information, the booklets actually encourage improvement efforts as hospitals compete for patient health care dollars.

Obviously, for care to be effective the patient has to understand his or her responsibility. Doctors have not always taken the time and trouble to explain

EXAMPLE: ORTHOPEDIC SURGERY

Patients vary a great deal. Those patients who require orthopedic surgery can benefit from standardized, multidisciplinary care that reinforces effective communication. Age and comorbidities have an impact on healing and recovery. Family support has an impact on postoperative care planning. Imagine two different patients who require hip replacement surgery. One patient is a young athlete who lives with his family and is in very good health and the other is an eighty-year-old in vulnerable health. Although their conditions and treatments may be similar, the two patients may require different levels of care, different involvement of staff, and different ancillary services and may also have quite different expectations for recovery. Those differences are more likely to be taken into account for both clinical and organizational planning when a team is involved in care.

Orthopedists use clinical guidelines with great success and embraced them before other disciplines took advantage of them, especially in hip replacement surgery, perhaps because although the actual implant is patient specific, the surgical procedure follows similar general outlines in all patients. The hip surgery itself is only part of the hospitalization; rehabilitation, which is highly dependent on the patient's willingness to cooperate, is critical for the outcome to be successful. Therefore it is important to orthopedic surgeons that their patients be educated about the procedure, be familiar with the expectations for recovery, and know what to anticipate posthospitalization.

To promote patient education in one hospital, nurses met with several patients at a time to answer questions, reassure them about the procedure and attempt to reduce their normal anxiety. The nurses talked about what to expect regarding anesthetics, recovery, and being on the hospital's surgical floor, as well as about the surgical procedure itself. Surgeons realized it was extremely important for patients to understand what to expect regarding pain and the importance of pain management to recovery. When communication was effective, patients were much more compliant with treatment, especially with the required physical therapy and pain management. Patients were also educated about getting assistance at home following discharge.

Over a period of time the surgical team developed a patient-friendly guideline to help surgical patients understand their plan of care (see Figure 3.3). Everything was outlined and explained: exercise, diet, special stockings, rehabilitation, and the importance of mobilization. Discharge instructions detailed what complications the patients should watch for and explained when to call the doctor. Patients were taught about observing their wounds and about the importance of walking and mobility for healing.

FIGURE 3.3 *Total hip replacement guideline, patient version*

TOTAL HIP REPLACEMENT GUIDELINE	
Patient Version	
This protocol is a general guideline and does not represent a professional care standard governing provider's obligation to patients. Care is revised to meet the individual patient's needs.	
BLOOD DRAWING	Blood work may be drawn by the Health Care team as ordered by the doctor. It may be necessary to draw blood several times during the day in order to check your condition
TESTS	Additional tests ma... explain any tests th...
TREATMENTS	You will have an i... triangle pillow) be... cross your legs. A ... removed before y... it will also be rem... hip, it will be chan... your bed, to make moving in bed easier. Inflatable cuffs may be placed around your legs while in bed to help the circulation.
MEDICATIONS	You may receive antibiotics through your intravenous line (I.V.) and you may receive medication to prevent blood clots. Your pain medication will be based on your needs, how it is given will be ordered by your doctor.
DIET	Your diet will be o... speak to you abou...
ACTIVITY	Your activity will b... You will be instruc... You will be seen b...
TEAM ACTIVITIES	Members of the H... questions that you...
EDUCATION	You will be taught... and manage your ... beign asked your n... team before you r... will be taught how to deep breathe and cough and use the incentive spirometer to keep your lungs clear. You will be taught about the medication you are taking and the possible side effects. You will also be taught hip precautions to help prevent dislocating your new hip and are advised to call for help before gettting out of bed. You will be taught the importance of not smoking and the effects of second hand smoke if needed.
DISCHARGE PLANNING	Your discharge plan will be based on your needs. If you have questions about home care or were receiving home care services please tell your nurse. A Social worket/Case manager may visit you to talk about your discharge plan. Your nurse will go over your discharge instructions with you and your family before you go home.

MEDICATIONS
You may receive antibiotics through your intravenous line (I.V.) and you may receive medication to prevent blood clots. Your pain medication will be based on your needs; how it is given will be ordered by your doctor.

DISCHARGE PLANNING
Your discharge plan will be based on your needs. If you have questions about home care or were previously receiving home care services please tell your nurse. A Social Worker/Case Manager may visit you to talk about your discharge plan. Your nurse will go over your discharge instructions with you and your family before you go home.

to their patients the importance of following instructions. Perhaps they assumed that nursing staff were taking care of patient education. But evidence indicates that both verbal and written communications are often not effective, at some physical cost to the patient and financial cost to the organization.

For example, if providing patients with discharge instructions is perceived as a task to be done to ensure compliance with the CMS measure that requires documentation of discharge instructions, the organization may receive financial incentives for compliance but there may be no added value for the patient. However, in an environment where the patient is the focus of the discharge instruction, effective education takes place about the importance of following medication, diet, and exercise instructions and keeping the initial posthospitalization appointment with the physician.

Effectively communicating discharge instructions results in improved health status for many patients. It is not sufficient simply to hand a list of medications and some scribbled notes to a patient upon discharge. Often patients are so eager to get out of the hospital that they do not even look at their discharge documents until they get home—when it's too late to ask for explanations. It is important that these instructions be explained before discharge and that patients have ample opportunity to ask questions about posthospitalization care. When patients leave the hospital without understanding their medication instructions or their follow-up care, they often end up back in the hospital or doctor's office. Effective communication helps them avoid unnecessary complications and extra physician visits.

When I was responsible for implementing a quality management program in a health care system, I focused on the patient and made use of a performance improvement methodology (Plan-Do-Check-Act, or PDCA) that involved organizational governance. By incorporating these leaders into the process, expectations were set for the organization. When I reviewed patient preparedness for surgery and admission to the hospital from the ED, I discovered that many of these patients were not informed, felt that they had poor communication with the clinicians, and were anxious and scared. Elderly patients who were transferred to the ED from nursing homes were not only ill, anxious, and scared but often disoriented and confused. Lack of time in the busy ED setting, lack of personnel to adequately prepare patients for their hospitalization, and the administrative goal of increasing volume resulted in patients being left to cope on their own. When these issues were brought to the attention of the organization's board members, they determined to fix the problem.

To help rectify this situation, I worked with the nursing staff to create patient-friendly pathways and informational guidelines that would educate and, we hoped, calm confused patients. Our experience indicated that when patients can anticipate what will occur they are less anxious and are more compliant with treatment. Information helps patients understand the importance of dietary restrictions, pain management, and ambulation. For example, a pneumonia pathway written for patients might explain the role of respiratory therapy for the patient, issues involved in pain management, and the importance of smoking cessation counseling (see Figure 3.4).

Patients are actually entitled to effective communication. The New York State Health Department, for example, has established guidelines for patient rights that require foreign language translators and sign language interpreters for patients who may need help communicating, and simplification of medical terminology so that laypeople can understand it. If patients can show that there

FIGURE 3.4 *Pneumonia guideline, patient version*

PNEUMONIA GUIDELINE
Patient Version

This protocol is a general guideline and does not represent a professional care standard governing provider's obligation to patients. Care is revised to meet the individual patient's needs.

BLOOD DRAWING	A member of the Health Care team may draw your blood as ordered by your doctor. It may be necessary to draw blood several times during the day in order to check your condition.
TESTS	Additional tests may be ordered by your doctor. The Health Care team will explain any tests that are ordered.
TREATMENTS	You will have an intravenous line (IV). You will have an abduction pillow (a firm triangle pillow) between your legs while you are in bed to remind you not to cross your legs. A tube will be placed in your bladder to drain urine, it will be removed before you go home. You may have a drain coming from your incision, it will also be removed before you go home. You will have a bandage over your hip, it will be changed ___ your bed, to make m___ your legs while in bed
MEDICATIONS	You may receive anti___ receive medication to ___ based on your needs,
DIET	Your diet will be orde___ speak to you about y___
ACTIVITY	Your activity will be ___ You will be instructed ___ You will be seen by a ___
TEAM ACTIVITIES	Members of the Heal___ questions that you or ___
EDUCATION	You will be taught h___ and manage your pain. You will be taught safety precautions, which will include beign asked your name and date of birth by the members of the Health Care team before you receive any medications, treatments, procedures or tests. You will be taught how to deep breathe and cough and use the incentive spirometer to keep your lungs clear. You will be taught about the medication you are taking and the possible side effects. You will also be taught hip precautions to help prevent dislocating your new hip and are advised to call for help before gettting out of bed. You will be taught the importance of not smoking and the effects of second hand smoke if needed.
DISCHARGE PLANNING	Your discharge plan will be based on your needs. If you have questions about home care or were receiving home care services please tell your nurse. A Social worket/Case manager may visit you to talk about your discharge plan. Your nurse will go over your discharge instructions with you and your family before you go home.

EDUCATION
You will be taught to use the pain scale. This will help staff to understand and manage your pain. You will be taught safety precautions, which will include being asked your name and date of birth by the members of the Health Care team before your receive any medications, treatments, procedures, or tests. You will be taught about the medications you are taking and any possible side effects. You will also be given advice/counseling on not smoking and the effects of secondhand smoke.

was failed communication and that they were not provided with appropriate translators, hospitals can be sued for large sums.

Caregivers should become sensitive to patients' level of literacy and language skills and also be aware of cultural habits that may have an impact on how information is interpreted. Health care organizations such as the Joint Commission, the CMS, the IHI, the Institute of Medicine, the AMA, the Agency for Healthcare Research and Quality (AHRQ), and health departments in various states have published patient literacy guidelines for health care professionals, hoping to alert caregivers to the reality that many of their patients may not have the literacy skills to understand medical instructions.

Low health literacy is commonplace and too often overlooked as an important factor in communicating information. People with a low level of literacy have trouble reading and understanding the front page of a newspaper or reading a bus schedule. Imagine how difficult it would be for them to comprehend informed consent forms or medication instructions. Low health literacy is understood to mean having difficulty with understanding vocabulary and using numbers at level that allows one to function effectively in a health care environment.

According to AHRQ, 90 million Americans scored at low literacy levels on the 1992 National Adult Literacy Survey. More recent data (2007), based on the AHRQ National Healthcare Disparities Report, revealed that only one in ten people had the literacy skills to manage their health. The AMA's Ad Hoc Committee on Health Literacy for the Council on Scientific Affairs has reported that low literacy leads to substandard medical care and adverse outcomes. Substandard care related to low literacy is encountered not only in the hospital setting but also in preventive care; AHRQ has found that preventive measures such as mammography screening, getting flu vaccines, or taking children for wellness visits are all linked to health literacy, with individuals with low literacy tending not to take advantage of preventive opportunities. Low literacy has serious health consequences for patients and financial consequences for health care organizations.

For everyone's benefit, patients need to be educated about their health status and care. Because many advantages arise from educating patients, CMS requires that hospitals devise processes for clear communication and patient education. For example, CMS and the Joint Commission require documentation that patients who smoke and have certain conditions (acute myocardial infarction or AMI, pneumonia) have received education on smoking cessation during their hospitalization. Compliance with this measure means that patients are taught; documenting this education results in financial rewards to the hospital. Although national guidelines recommend smoking cessation counseling because research shows that patients who smoke and who receive such education are more likely than noneducated patients to quit smoking, these recommendations were rarely met. Therefore CMS has introduced the financial incentive. Through measures the government is trying to influence patient education and improve care—that is, promote value in health care.

National agencies such as the Hospital Quality Alliance, which is a collaboration of many organizations—including organizations that represent hospitals and also such groups as the AMA, the American Heart Association, the Joint Commission, and the CMS—are also providing an impetus for improving communication through initiatives that measure effective communication. Participating hospital organizations measure how many patients actually received appropriate discharge instructions, for example. Another measure that helps to evaluate the effectiveness of communication is readmission rates for patients with chronic diseases. A readmission may indicate that treatment the first time around was ineffective or that the patient had a poor understanding of follow-up treatment. Research shows that failure to attend adequately to the care transition at discharge from the hospital results in additional annual Medicare spending of $15 billion.

NEAR-MISS REPORTING

Health care organizations are attempting to improve communication and avoid errors through specialized techniques and tools that directly promote effective and efficient care. One example of such a technique is developing a near-miss, or good-catch, program.

Near misses occur all the time in hospitals. For example, a nurse might see that another nurse is about to administer the incorrect medication and she or he intervenes to correct the potential error. Harm is averted by the intervention.

Documenting near misses is important because everyone on the health care team is then made aware of what might have happened if the error had reached the patient. The Joint Commission and state departments of health recommend collecting data on near misses for precisely this reason: when you know what could go wrong, you can take steps to make sure it doesn't go wrong. But collecting data on near misses has proved problematic. Caregivers are frequently reluctant to admit their mistakes, especially those which could have resulted in a serious incident. Caregivers do not want to be shamed about their caregiving in front of their peers. Also, many caregivers do not even recognize quick corrections as near misses.

Imagine walking down an icy walkway and slipping and almost turning your ankle. Because you did not actually injure yourself, you might ignore the momentary incident completely. However, if you were looking for areas of danger to yourself, you might recognize the slip as an opportunity to learn something. You might recognize a need to avoid icy walkways, to have salt or other material put on walkways to improve traction, to change footgear, or to have signs put out asking people to use extra caution. However, if you simply walk on, there is no opportunity to learn anything from the event.

There are steps that have been proved effective in lowering the barriers that keep people from reporting near misses. One way to avoid shame and blame is to ensure anonymous reporting. Another technique is to classify the near misses into categories so that what might otherwise be dismissed as

NEAR MISS   A near miss is defined as an event that *almost* occurred. If the event had occurred, it would have caused harm to a patient.

unimportant is defined. For example, Figure 3.5 shows a distribution of near misses collected from a hospital's operating room (OR) nurses. Such a distribution can explain to caregivers the scope and significance of certain problem areas. The largest category is labeled "multiple near misses," meaning that a single patient faced potential harm in several areas. For example, an incorrect patient ID band may lead to other problems, such as medication errors or even wrong-site surgery. Another problem area in this distribution involves informed consent. Efforts to ensure completed informed consent prior to surgery have been made for years. Yet clearly, according to these data, problems still exist. Near-miss data should be collected and reported out to performance improvement groups for discussion and improvement efforts. Aggregating data about near misses allows organizations to identify gaps in safety.

Accurate patient identification is crucial for safe and appropriate care. Through the near-miss program for which the data shown in Figure 3.5 were gathered, the nursing staff identified a problem that if not resolved could have resulted in serious patient harm. Analysis showed that patients who were being prepared for surgery were given ID bands that became illegible when they came into contact with liquid. Once this issue was identified, this potentially high-risk, high-volume problem was addressed. Bands were changed, at low cost, and patient safety improved.

Another useful method for encouraging near-miss reporting is to make available real-time reports, perhaps through a Web-based technology. Once a caregiver moves on to other chores, it is difficult to remember to report an incident that had no impact on the patient. However, if there is a mechanism readily available that enables the caregiver to report quickly and anonymously,

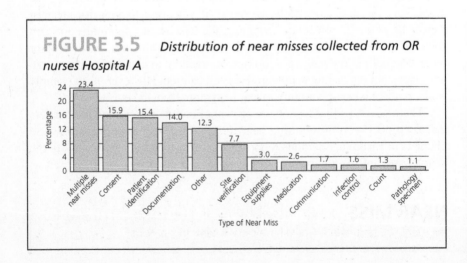

FIGURE 3.5   *Distribution of near misses collected from OR nurses Hospital A*

rates of reports improve. In our health system we introduced a Web-based anonymous near-miss reporting system, and the volume of near-miss reports increased dramatically.

CHRONIC DISEASE MANAGEMENT

Chronic diseases, such as diabetes, asthma, and heart disease, are the most prevalent, expensive, and preventable health problems. Every year almost 2 million Americans die of chronic diseases, accounting for 70 percent of all deaths in the United States. According to the CMS, medical care for patients with chronic disease accounts for more than 75 percent of the $2 trillion we spend annually on medical care.

Clearly, it is in everyone's interest to learn how to best manage chronic disease. Poor management increases hospital expenses unnecessarily, whereas good management has clinical, financial, and organizational rewards. If a patient's condition is not managed properly and the condition deteriorates, the patient typically ends up in ICU care, among the most expensive and resource-intensive units in a hospital. If the patient has a flare-up of a chronic condition, it usually means there are complications, which may involve many specialists.

If a patient with heart failure, for example, ends up in the ICU, an intensivist or a hospitalist has to communicate with the primary physician about the treatment plan. Often, poor coordination among the various specialists results in a longer LOS than would otherwise be necessary and inappropriate uses of resources because no one is responsible for managing the flow of information and services. Nurses frequently complain about the time consumed in filling out the paperwork necessary for documenting individual patients' treatment plans; they claim it takes them away from the more important clinical care they need to perform. Maybe so, but someone has to coordinate, communicate, and document patient care for it to be effective and efficient.

An especially vulnerable period in the patient care cycle comes between the time the physician signs the discharge order and the time the patient actually departs. During this period, which may run as long as twenty-four or even forty-eight hours, patients still require medication, nutrition, perhaps physical assistance, and information about medication reconciliation. Typically, however, nursing staff are busy with incoming patients, and it is easy to neglect outgoing ones. Hospitals have realized, through measures, that readmittance rates are increased when discharged patients are not included in the daily treatment regime.

With the aging of the population, managing chronic illnesses such as diabetes and heart failure at home is essential if the resources of health care institutions are not to be overextended. New technologies, such as

EXAMPLE: IMPROVING DISEASE MANAGEMENT BY IMPROVING COMMUNICATION

In my experience, many patients with congestive heart failure (CHF) are elderly (over seventy-five years old) and require multiple medications to manage their health. This medication is often increased during a hospitalization, sometimes doubling between admission and discharge. Elderly patients who require many medications run the risk of mismanaging their treatment unless they have clear and explicit education.

In an attempt to optimize outcomes for CHF patients and to ensure that care is continued beyond the hospitalization, I train residents in how to provide simple and intelligible discharge instructions, materials, and protocols. I have them review random charts retrospectively to assess the effectiveness of the patients' discharge instructions. The reason discharge instructions are so important for heart failure patients is that managing the disease at home can prevent hospital readmission and avoid crises. Details of appropriate diet and the importance of exercising, taking medication reliably, and arranging follow-up care with physicians are all outlined in discharge instructions.

During this training process the residents found problems with discharge instruction legibility and that patients had difficulty in decoding physicians' medication orders. They also discovered that many patients took double their dose of prescribed medication because they had not been adequately educated about generic medicines. Thinking that a generic was a different medication from a trade name medication they were familiar with, patients would take both. Furthermore, many patients did not realize that it was their responsibility to follow up with their physician after being released from the hospital. Also, patients were not educated about reasons for them to return to the ED.

The residents realized that the discharge form required revision in order to make it easier to understand; that the purpose of medications had to be described in simple, lay terms; that efforts were needed to ensure there was no duplication of generic and trade name drugs; that to ensure effective follow-up, a communication line should be established between the hospital and the patient's primary care physician; and that attention needed to be given to reconciling medication before and after a hospital admission. The result of these improvements would be better patient understanding of personal medical conditions and treatments and decreased readmissions. A little thought and effort can make a huge difference in patient care and organizational efficiency.

telemedicine, are increasingly being used both to educate patients about home management of their conditions and to reduce expensive home health visits. This technology allows chronic conditions to be monitored via computer and TV screens. Our experience at the North Shore-LIJ Health System home care services shows that patients who are monitored more frequently have better outcomes and that virtual monitoring can be just as effective as actual nursing visits.

Educating patients about medication and clarifying discharge instructions involves very little financial outlay. What it does require is acculturation of the clinical staff to a patient-focused environment. Because treating chronic disease is very expensive for hospitals, and dealing with patients in crisis who require the ICU is expensive as well, it is to everyone's benefit to educate patients about managing their chronic diseases.

TASK FORCES

To change physician attitudes and to promote a patient-focused environment, hospitals can use the multidisciplinary task force to develop methods of improved communication that create staff buy-in for new processes and procedures. This task force should explicitly articulate its charge and detail the benefits that are expected from the improvement efforts (see Table 3.2).

Task forces can also become responsible for initiating and maintaining constant feedback about the success of new programs. For example, if you devise a program for smoking cessation education for CHF patients, a task force can help in developing methods and personnel for program implementation. Informational booklets can be designed and given to each patient.

This task force should include everyone involved in working with CHF patients and be led by a prominent physician. It should devise measures, with

TABLE 3.2   **Quality management and evidence-based task forces**

Charge	Benefits
Provide understanding, direction, and tools to achieve improved processes and outcomes.	Optimize patient care Standardize measures Share best practices Identify gaps in safe patient care Improve clinical involvement Enhance communication

TABLE 3.3   **Heart failure clinical pathway**

Interventions	Outcomes
Nutrition consult	O₂ sat is >90%
Chest X-ray	Ejection fraction is documented
EKG	Free from weight gain
Pulse oximetry	Tolerates activity level
Daily weights	Understands dietary regime
If ejection fraction is <40% use digoxin, diuretics, and ACEI [ACE inhibitor] unless contraindicated	Participates in ADLs [activities of daily living] within limits of physiological tolerance
Activity as prior to admission	Coumadin at discharge if Afib
If ejection fraction is <40% discharge on ACEI unless contraindicated	Written discharge instructions given
Coumadin (if Afib [atrial fibrillation])	Educated on smoking cessation
Discharge	

explicit numerators and denominators, that increase understanding of the value of meeting the program expectations and should develop consensus about how to implement the measures in practice. Usually nurses are trained to collect data, but physicians have to remain accountable and responsible for oversight of the data collection process.

Embedding the measures in a clinical pathway or guideline is useful because data can then be recorded using a Web-based tool and can become part of the medical record. Table 3.3 lists the interventions and outcomes noted on a pathway for heart failure treatment, reminding caregivers about what interventions are expected and what appropriate outcomes should be.

Another advantage to embedding measures in the pathway is that the data collected are formatted for demonstrating compliance with CMS standards, a piece of organizational efficiency. Quality management research analysts analyze such data for rates of compliance and can target areas of noncompliance for improvements. Measures are used as baselines. When there is variation from the measure, then the practitioner needs to explain why the measure was not met. In other words, CMS measures force physicians to look at their performance and compare it to the performance of the rest of the nation.

PATIENT RIGHTS AND RESPONSIBILITIES

Anyone interacting with health care in the past few years has been made aware of HIPAA (Health Insurance Portability and Accountability Act) regulations. These are rules put into effect by the federal government to promote patient privacy and empower patients to control who gets medical information about them. Although the regulations are cumbersome and somewhat maddening to many health care professionals, the goal was to help establish a patient-focused environment for information. Under HIPAA patients are encouraged to voice their concerns and complaints to appropriate staff and organizations. Health care organizations usually have a department that processes patient complaints, and state departments of health and the Joint Commission are also repositories for complaints. Families and patients have the opportunity to complain about inadequate or substandard care and very often do so—not because they want recompense in a malpractice suit, but because they want their concerns to be heard and they want something in the organization to change to better protect patient safety.

This is a new culture, one in which the patient oversees the actions of the caregivers, monitoring whether the caregiver washed his or her hands and whether the patient's medication conforms to what was ordered. Many patients find they need to remind staff about their nutritional needs and restrictions. Patients with diabetes should be on low-sugar diets, for example, and when a tray appears with pie and ice cream, the patient has to know there will be health consequences and that staff need to be made aware of the error.

The move toward transparency focuses on the patient knowing what has occurred—including mistakes and errors. Clinicians are required to admit mistakes and inform patients about their care. This is a new paradigm: the patient has the right to know. Constant and clear communication is expected to be documented in the treatment plan.

Hospitals have ethics committees staffed by clinicians who can help patients with difficult decisions, especially those related to end-of-life care. Many hospitals make available to the community educational workshops and seminars about living wills, advance directives, and powers of attorney so that patients coming into the hospital already have an understanding of their rights. In 1990, Congress passed the Patient Self-Determination Act, which ensures that patients participate in their treatment decisions. Advance directives and living wills can be used for guidance when patients are too ill or incompetent to make important decisions in real time. The idea is that the patient's wishes be honored.

COMPASSIONATE CARING

Good communication is based on trust. When the caregiver is perceived as caring and compassionate, the patient is more eager to offer personal and private information than he or she would be otherwise. The more effective the communication, the less likely it is that the patient will be harmed. Therefore, good communication and compassionate care help to improve patient safety. In a health care environment the participants are unequal; a helpless, ill, frightened patient is entirely dependent on caregivers to provide a safe environment and to help him or her. With such inequality, the responsibility for effective communication resides with the caregiver.

Compassionate caregivers are more effective than others because they can elicit a more detailed and complete patient history and make a better assessment of the patient's health status. For these reasons, for the first time, medical students are being taught effective communication techniques. They need to know how to listen carefully and respectfully. They need to be aware of their patients' understanding of their instructions. Clinicians are trained to use science to evaluate disease, and are also encouraged to use art in the form of their experience and instinct in providing medical care. Introducing the notion of art into the science of medicine supports subjectivity in an otherwise objective method of medical analysis. By adding compassion to this interplay between objectivity and subjectivity, the medical professional improves patient care.

EXAMPLE: COMPASSIONATE CARE— REDUCING RESTRAINTS

In an effort to increase humane practice and meet the personal needs of patients, the Joint Commission and CMS view the use of restraints as poor care and encourage alternatives that reduce use of restraints. Restraints are used for agitated patients, patients who are not compliant or who are disruptive, or patients at high risk for falls. Proper communication helps to obviate the need for restraints, as does increased staffing and monitoring.

In one of the North Shore-LIJ Health System's nursing homes, the CEO, Dennis Connors, determined to reduce restraints on patients who were at high risk for falls. He made it a point to visibly engage with staff, communicating his commitment, and was on the floor and at the bedside of the patients often. Usually administrators do not venture out to the patient units, but such a commitment sends a powerful message to the staff. This compassionate CEO spoke not only with the clinicians involved in patient care but also with housekeeping, security, and nurses aides—everyone who had access to the patients.

He asked them all to call a nurse if they saw anyone getting out of bed alone. He made staff part of the treatment team. He brought everyone together and explained why observation was so important. By enlisting help from the entire staff, he sensitized them all on the risk for falls and their role in prevention. Restraint use was reduced as was the incidence of falls. Such a simple and powerful intervention: talk to the staff.

Providing compassionate care is a challenge in the overcrowded conditions and with the low staffing ratios that most health care workers experience. Organizations can and should develop processes that compensate for these conditions. Not only does the patient benefit from compassionate care but the organization does as well. Falls, decubitus ulcers (pressure injuries), aspiration pneumonia, and other unnecessary complications can be reduced when the focus of care changes toward proactively preventing problems. Often the importance of compassion is overlooked or even disparaged, as in the attitude that says, "Don't get too involved; it might affect your objectivity." To the contrary, I tell the caregivers I teach to get involved and to care as much as they can. Talk to patients as if they were friends or loved ones. Be sensitive to their emotional and psychological state. Try to diminish the power differential between caregiver and patient.

If the patient is at the end-of-life stage, with do not resuscitate (DNR) orders, the caregiving team should assess the patient's appropriateness for hospice care. Such patients require treatment different from that given to patients in crisis in the OR, for example. End-of-life patients may require someone to discuss options with the family and to be present and compassionate with the patient. These techniques are also part of good medical care. Also, a patient who is depressed or suicidal will rarely articulate his or her emotional state to a resident taking a history and physical. But in a patient-centered environment, the doctor becomes a keen observer who might detect symptoms and call for consultation.

SUMMARY

A patient-focused environment promotes improved outcomes through

- Increasing communication between patient and caregiver

- Coordinating care among caregivers across the continuum

- Educating patients about and involving patients in their treatment and care

- Improving efficiency in disease management

- Standardizing communication processes (with techniques such as SBAR)

- Proactively anticipating risks to patient safety (with analyses such as FMEA)

- Using clinical pathways to coordinate and standardize treatment

- Ensuring that patients understand their discharge instructions

- Sensitizing caregivers to issues involved in patient education

- Encouraging near-miss reporting of potential gaps in safety
- Promoting a team approach for caregivers
- Increasing transparency

KEY TERMS

clinical guideline   health literacy
clinical pathway   near misses
communication   patient education
handoff   task force

THINGS TO THINK ABOUT

Imagine that an elderly patient suffering from congestive heart failure is admitted to the emergency department from a local nursing home. Address the communication flow at all stages of care:

1. At what points is information transferred?

2. What are the potential barriers to effective communication?

3. What are effective strategies to overcome these barriers?

4. How should the patient be involved in his or her care?

5. What data would you use to ensure that the patient is treated effectively?

CHAPTER

4

UNDERSTANDING PROCESSES, OUTCOMES, AND COSTS

LEARNING OBJECTIVES

- Understand the concept of never events
- Describe the connections among waste, good outcomes, and efficiency
- Describe how the PDCA cycle can improve outcomes
- Describe the value of clinical pathways in improving organizational efficiency
- Discuss issues related to end-of-life care in terms of processes, outcomes, and costs

In the previous chapters I have discussed how some processes lead to negative outcomes and how taking steps toward prevention results in improvements for the patient and for the hospital. (This topic is examined in detail in my book *Measuring Health Care*.) In this chapter I focus on the ways in which external agencies are leading the movement to reduce negative outcomes by institutionalizing expectations for prevention, and the ways in which hospitals are responding to these changes.

SOME EVENTS SHOULD NEVER OCCUR

In defining certain occurrences as "never events," the Centers for Medicare and Medicaid Services (CMS) has focused attention on patient safety issues. The concept of the never event targets outcomes that are preventable and should never happen, such as patient falls, serious pressure injuries, surgeries on the wrong site, blood transfusion reactions caused by the administration of incorrect blood types, and foreign objects left in surgery patients. These events cause great harm to patients and cost hospitals and insurers large sums of money as they deal with the health consequences of these errors.

Several states have passed legislation requiring hospitals to report never events, and the CMS has a never event program that encourages hospitals to develop programs to eliminate such outcomes through deliberate preventive strategies. The hope is that by publishing negative outcomes resulting from these events and lowering reimbursement for care related to preventable errors, these errors will be reduced. However, changing behavior is a slow process, and most hospitals have not yet met the national benchmarks for establishing preventive programs, ones that would result, for example, in no falls. It is interesting to examine the reasons for this delay, because the benefit to both patient and hospital is obvious. One explanation is that prevention efforts require a cultural change that overcomes organizational barriers and that establishing a new culture takes resources and time.

Through its never event program CMS is trying to teach administrators and clinicians about the relationship between improving patient outcomes and increasing reimbursement, that is, the link between quality and finance. Today, quality variables must be added to the economic definition of care because a hospital that does not reduce or prevent never events might not receive payment for treatment of those events. The idea behind the CMS program is that the health care organization's CEO, faced with financial pressure, will promote good processes and develop preventive strategies. Because of financial pressure, leaders will begin to take an active role in developing programs to prevent, monitor, and improve on the quality indicators set by the CMS.

Traditionally, chief financial officers (CFOs) and chief medical officers (CMOs) hear about never events or poor outcomes from accreditation organizations and state departments of health through their ongoing surveys. Senior administrators usually do not interact with caregivers or quality management functions in ways that would help them to understand the relationship between the delivery of care and poor outcomes. Often, they do not realize the financial

EXAMPLE: SPECIALTY BEDS

One of the challenges for modern health care organizations is to introduce change and define outcomes based on measures. When I explain to physicians, for example, that their patients' sepsis is the result of decubitus ulcers (or decubiti), I need to show them data. I have to convince them that yes, *their* patients have infection, not just the patients in some random sample from another (inferior) organization. Once confronted with data about their patients, they give me their attention. Then the question becomes why do their patients get decubiti? Did some part of the care process break down, or was the issue one of clinician competency, poor assessment, or perhaps inadequate equipment, such as the lack of specialty beds?

Hospitals purchase expensive specialty beds to reduce decubiti: the investment pays for itself if it lowers the rate and severity of these injuries. To link the quality and financial variables of such purchases, a savvy CFO would involve quality management professionals who could research the usefulness of specialty beds to the patients and do a cost-benefit analysis of the purchase of such products.

Medical care, as I have suggested previously, tends to be more reactive than proactive. Specialty beds (and other useful equipment) often reside in storage and are doled out only after serious decubiti have occurred. So even though the organization buys the beds, they are not used appropriately to prevent decubiti in high-risk patients. Every day that a specialty bed goes unused is a day in which the purchase or rental price of the bed is wasted. Improvement has to occur at the source of the problem, not just as a response to the end product of poor processes.

To understand the financial and health implications of specialty beds, data are required. To integrate purchasing and quality requires that finance committees think outside their traditional boxes. The CFO should enlist the organization's quality management department to gather information about how the beds are used, how often, on which units, and with what outcomes. Data could be gathered comparing the outcomes of patients put on specialty beds against the outcomes of patients who are not. The CFO should ask the frontline workers if the beds or other products add value to the staff and patients. To improve both clinical care and financial success, the CEO should go to the patient units and demand explanations for the incidence of decubiti in patients. He or she should participate in meetings of quality performance improvement committees with the CMO and CFO and help to develop appropriate steps to reduce negative outcomes from these (and other) preventable injuries.

impact of poor outcomes nor do they understand the financial implications of efficient processes.

LEADERS' ROLE IN GOOD OUTCOMES

Senior leaders need to learn the value of connecting bedside care, patient outcomes, and cost. Because the CFO is the person most responsible for educating members of the board of trustees about the financial picture of the organization, the finance committee of the board (the group that makes the highest level financial decisions) must be educated about the importance of linking quality to finance and of taking steps to reduce waste.

Health care reformers talk about increasing the efficiency of care, and efficiency is usually defined as short length of stay (LOS). However, another and productive way to define efficiency is through the concept of waste. If waste is reduced, efficiency is increased. If waste is reduced, then unnecessary expenditure is also reduced. Waste reduction promotes cost savings. Waste is actually a better measure of efficiency than LOS or utilization because the focus is on a particular process, procedure, or disease.

Waste reduction is based on quality outcomes; waste indicators are integrally related to quality indicators. If the CFO and CEO look at these waste indicators rather than the traditional variables of volume and LOS, they would consider decubiti rates and other preventable outcomes, such as falls and infections, as waste indicators. Never events are wasteful. Ideally, the governing board's quality committee and finance committee should merge and become a single entity, looking at care from both dimensions. Reducing waste improves care—and improves financial margins.

For example, the cost of falls in terms of waste can be measured and tracked over time. A measure can be developed where, for instance, the numerator is the number of malpractice claims for falls and the denominator is the total number of falls. The higher the ratio of claims per falls, the bigger the financial deficit for the budget. Instituting a falls prevention program may or may not improve the situation. This measure will expose flaws in the changed processes. Unless there is a commitment to corrective actions, simply developing prevention programs will not work.

When leaders focus on waste reduction, they must also establish a strong infrastructure for quality management. Health care leadership would do well to take a lesson from former General Electric CEO and chairman Jack Welch, who believed that cost, quality, and service were interrelated and that to succeed in business an organization had to eliminate waste and enhance quality and communication. By combining these three forces, GE provided better value to the public. The product would be without defects (eliminating waste), and the profit margin would increase. There are very few maverick CEOs leading health care organizations. However, the most successful understand the value of incorporating quality management methods, identifying weak points in the provision of care, initiating change and improvement, and focusing on good outcomes and waste reduction.

The role of the board of trustees in hospitals is to provide effective checks and balances about performance. Board members need to take their oversight responsibility seriously and understand why compliance with evidence-based measures results in organizational and clinical improvements. Once they become educated in quality management philosophy, they can understand the connection between cost, waste, outcomes, and profit. Reports should contain the full scope of finance and quality measures together. Only through introducing quality into financial reports will the organization improve and change. The artificial division between administrative and clinical concerns should be bridged.

Incorporating evidence-based medicine into standardized care minimizes waste because doing so creates consistency. The CMS approach in the pay-for-performance initiative has attempted to eliminate subjective decisions in favor of objective standards through requiring compliance with evidence-based indicators of treatment for various diagnoses, such as pneumonia or heart failure. By eliminating variation, waste is reduced. Clinicians can plan for care proactively and prospectively; the formulary for medications and equipment should be developed on the basis of population, rather than individual patients; staffing can be efficiently planned, and patients can move through the continuum more efficiently when processes are standardized and consistent.

The Joint Commission requires that leaders be involved in quality, but again the regulatory requirement is often perceived as a compliance issue rather than an impetus for improvement. Until and unless the senior leadership gets involved in improvements, things will remain the same. Involvement means that the CEO addresses quality management in weekly administrative meetings. Quality, organizational, and economic variables should be linked for optimal performance.

The historical division between clinical care and administrative responsibility is antiquated in today's marketplace. These functions, traditionally isolated from each other, have to be merged. Administrators need to learn about the delivery of clinical care and physicians need to become accountable for organizational improvements such as moving patients safely through the continuum of care or complying with evidence-based indicators for increased reimbursement.

When the CEO gets behind a program, it has a better chance of success than it would if leadership commitment were lacking. For example, in one hospital when a family complained about a patient acquiring a pressure injury while hospitalized and threatened to sue for malpractice, the CEO participated in the root cause analysis with the clinicians involved in the patient's care. The CEO wanted to understand what had happened and to ensure that new processes were developed that would prevent future occurrences. Once these programs are on the CEO's radar, and staff know about it, change occurs more readily than it would if the CEO had not gotten involved. An involved and participating CEO also encourages middle managers to be more accountable for the performance of their staffs and to be responsible for the impact of poor outcomes on the budget as well as on patient care.

However, very few CEOs feel comfortable changing practices. The arguments about how to achieve compliance (with electronic medical records or with additional nurses to review compliance, for example) can seem endless. Once the CEO understands that the issue is not compliance but improvement, the organization will become ripe for change.

For change to take place the CEO needs to embrace the quality management focus on evaluating weaknesses and strengths in the delivery of care. Many leaders have realized that they need to know the ropes of their own business from the bottom up, so to speak. Leaders should be encouraged to take this hands-on approach, to go visit the patient care units, talk to the kitchen staff, talk to people in the operating room (OR) locker room. The message gets clearly relayed that everyone is important, that the job everyone is doing is worth noticing, and that everyone's problems are relevant. This is a way to improve communication and to introduce change. It is a very different approach from sitting behind a desk in a closed office where entry is by invitation only.

PHYSICIANS' ROLE IN GOOD OUTCOMES

Physicians also need to incorporate quality variables into their delivery of care, and for physicians, just as for health care organizations, money provides a powerful incentive for change. Governmental agencies such as CMS are attempting to influence physician practice by offering financial rewards for compliance with evidence-based quality indicators. Physicians who are reluctant to change what they see as tried-and-true ways of practicing medicine may be loathe to incorporate, for example, the evidence that giving antibiotics to pneumonia patients within four hours of admission is the appropriate clinical intervention. However, with the incentive of a financial reward for complying with this variable, more physicians are incorporating such practice into their delivery of care.

Defining problems as things that are wrong with a process and that can be identified and improved requires a different mind-set from attempting to resolve every problem by tackling it at the individual patient level. It is easy to berate the nursing staff for not turning a bedridden patient often enough to avoid a pressure injury, for example, but data show that such an approach does not lead to improvements. It is more useful to think about problems from a process point of view or a patient population point of view (what problems typically arise?) or from the continuum point of view (what are the postsurgical goals for recovery?), and to work to develop treatment plans that link processes with outcomes.

However, many physicians give only lip service to data and distinguish between documenting compliance with an evidence-based measure and actually understanding its value. A physician's assistant or nurse is often assigned the responsibility for documentation, but ideally, these measures should encourage doctors to look at disease in a different way. If physicians define their delivery of care as part of a process, with data from aggregated populations, they have a different perspective than they have when they view a single patient during a single episode of care. If physicians look at a disease along the entire continuum of care, they consider the entire hospital experience.

For example, if a pneumonia patient receives antibiotics within four hours of admission, the doctor can anticipate a normal course of treatment and a predictable LOS. If there are no complicating factors, the patient will be changed from IV to oral medication on day 3 and be discharged on day 5. CMS variables help physicians define care as part of a continuum, a perspective that is extremely useful for organizational planning. In addition, the CMS indicators force physicians to include prevention as part of their normal course of treatment. The pneumonia patient is supposed to receive education on smoking cessation before discharge.

Physician behavior can also be influenced by bad publicity. For example, in an attempt to reduce unnecessary deaths, New York State collected data on coronary artery bypass graft (CABG) mortality. The data were risk adjusted to ensure valid comparisons among organizations. The state department of health focused on reducing mortality as a goal and required organizations to collect data on infection rates and reoperations. The department also developed measures for optimal care, such as giving beta blockers preoperatively and at discharge, and pressured health care organizations to comply with these measures. If a patient was excluded from the standard treatment, physicians were expected to explain the reason for the exclusion. When physicians complied with the measures, mortality decreased. Those physicians who still had higher than average mortality rates could no longer claim that their patients were sicker than comparable populations because the data proved the contrary. Those physicians had a choice: to improve their proficiency through education, to change their practice based on evidence, or to leave this specialized field of medicine.

Changing the process of care made a difference, although many doctors were initially skeptical that it would. They complied simply because not doing so would result in censure by the state. However, when the data showed that the outcomes were indeed improved, that mortality was reduced, clinicians began to change and came to believe that the measures were useful for more than compliance.

Encouraging physicians to participate on task forces can help to inculcate measures into daily care. When one of the North Shore-LIJ Health System hospitals determined to improve the outcomes of pneumonia patients, rather than review charts, quality management leaders developed a task force of the clinicians and staff involved in caring for this patient population. Our hope was that clinician involvement would encourage increased buy-in for developing measures and enforcing changed practices.

It was also an opportunity to educate clinicians about measures. We did not impose measures on them but asked them to develop criteria for best practices as well as appropriate inclusion and exclusion criteria for patient treatment. By proactively determining specific interventions that the task force members agreed would result in the best outcomes for patients, clinicians began to see the value of collecting data and reporting out results. The goal was to correlate certain variables with LOS, infection, and mortality rates.

Through data and with quality management professionals who worked alongside clinicians to establish improvements, physicians acknowledged problems and helped to devise solutions. Participating in such endeavors is a different way to think about medical care for many physicians, but success in terms of improved patient outcomes and improved financial outcomes reward this changed approach to care.

FINANCIAL VALUE OF GOOD OUTCOMES

Insurance companies understand the link between quality and cost and see the value of promoting good outcomes. They encourage changed practices by reducing malpractice insurance for hospitals that can document (with data) that they have standardized processes and good outcomes.

For example, according to Endurance Specialty Insurance Ltd., if a hospital can document that it meets the National Patient Safety Goals established by the Joint Commission (see Chapter Five), it is awarded 10 points. If the hospital meets the CMS measures and exceeds the national average by 5 percent, it is awarded another 10 points. If the hospital accumulates 90 points, it receives a 5 percent discount on insurance (see Figure 4.1). That

FIGURE 4.1 *Insurers discount for quality*

Leapfrog Group practices—meets all standards	**10**
Magnet status (American Nurses Association)	**10**
Healthgrades' Distinguished Hospital Award for patient safety or clinical excellence	**10**
CMS Core Measures compliance at 5% over national norm	**10**
Meeting Joint Commission's National Patient Safety Goals	**10**
IHI 5M Lives Campaign participant	**10**
US News & World Report's "America's Best Hospitals" recognition	**10**
Insured choice	**20**
TOTAL	**90**

Premium Credit Grading Scale

Points	Premium Credit
80–90	5%
70–79	4%
60–69	3%
50–59	2%
10–49	1%

Premium of $50,000,000 could receive
credit of $500,000 – $2,500,000

Source: Endurance Specialty Insurance Ltd.

number translates into millions of saved dollars. Such savings grab administrators' attention. These external influences are helping to teach the C suite that finance and quality are interrelated and that quality variables should be included in financial reports.

Managed care companies are also rewarding hospitals that can document improved outcomes and compliance with specific measures of care, through the pay-for-performance initiative. Blue Cross Blue Shield, for example, looks at cardiac surgery outcomes. It not only examines rates of risk-adjusted mortality but also collects data on readmission rates. Readmission is a quality variable as well as an organizational one because if a patient needs to be readmitted within a specific time frame it may indicate that the patient had inadequate care during the previous hospitalization or inadequate discharge instructions or procedures. For those organizations that can show improved rates of these variables, there is a financial reward.

All these efforts to incorporate safety and quality into the business of health care are not surprising. Health care, like other businesses, is financially driven, and what makes good health sense makes good financial sense. The surprising idea is that this connection has been made only recently—thanks to the external agencies that are insisting on compliance with quality measures. With money at stake, and the C suite committed to improvements, change is more likely to occur.

CHANGING THE TRADITIONAL CULTURE

The role of quality management has to be strengthened in health care organizations. The successful use of data and measures to define gaps in care and develop improvements can best be accomplished by professionals who examine data objectively. Quality management oversees quality. Unfortunately, health care organizations have been reducing most quality management to having nurses examine medical records for documentation of compliance with government regulatory measures. But when quality care is linked to financial rewards and when the goal of patient safety is linked to quality measures, the role of quality expands from compliance to improvement and to changing practice at the bedside. By being proactive and studying processes for flaws, by developing initiatives to collect data and monitor changed practices for improvements, and by using data analysts and statisticians to determine patterns and trends in outcomes, quality management can convince clinical and administrative leaders that change is necessary and desirable.

Transparency is another new concept that is taking root. Physicians are realizing that in order to survive in a competitive marketplace they need to have good results on publicly reported measures of quality and patient safety. An educated health care consumer demands good results. If results are not excellent, patients go elsewhere.

Before they can create a new health care culture, care providers have to become convinced that care without defects is efficient and effective care. The notion that certain complications are to be expected suggests that defects are tolerable. But when quality outcomes become the goal and the reduction of defects is central to care processes, there will be much greater patient safety, satisfaction, and financial success for the organization. Final accountability for changing the culture resides with the board and the CEO. Leadership has to lead the way.

The next phase in changing the health care culture will include evaluating care by examining process variables. CMS is introducing the concept of looking at medical diagnosis across the whole continuum of care, rather than focusing solely on the acute phase. Examining the entire process of care allows key risk points for the patient to be identified. For example, two vulnerable areas for patients are in the emergency department (ED) and at discharge. Developing measures to improve outcomes in both of these areas increases patient safety. If the organization is committed to complying with these measures, then the caregiver is, for example, focused on triage in the ED because the timing of antibiotic administration needs to be documented for compliance and financial rewards. A quick diagnosis means that there must be efficient and effective communication among services, such as between the ED clinicians and the radiology and laboratory staff. In addition to speeding up sluggish processes, such a focus results in patients with infections getting their appropriate interventions quickly. Everyone benefits from complying with evidence-based indicators.

On the other end of the care spectrum, at discharge, patients need to be effectively educated about their medication and follow-up care. Including post-discharge instructions in the provision of care (a practice encouraged by financial rewards for documenting that medication reconciliation has occurred or smoking cessation education has been given) improves patients' health and avoids unnecessary and wasteful complications and readmissions. Improved quality is reflected in improved patient outcomes. Improved patient outcomes are the result of relating process variables and outcomes.

Establishing a Method to Improve Outcomes

Through quality management tools, such as the Plan-Do-Check-Act (PDCA) cycle of performance improvement, processes can be examined and data collected and analyzed to target areas where improvement is necessary. The PDCA methodology focuses on identifying specific processes that are resulting in problems; it also establishes the probability of recurrence. Once the faulty process is identified, steps can be taken to improve it.

The PDCA cycle involves constantly prioritizing and reprioritizing areas for improvement based on data and the organization's goals. Collecting data about a problem or process identifies a baseline from which improvements can be measured. Once one or more improvements have been developed, through consensus and expert task forces, measurements to ascertain their effectiveness can be defined. Analyzing the data over time reveals whether each improvement is robust and successfully integrated into the delivery of

EXAMPLE: VENTILATORS One of the complications that may occur for patients on ventilators is ventilator-associated pneumonia, a condition identified by the Institute for Healthcare Improvement as one that hospitals should target for improvement efforts in order to reduce the rate of these pneumonias. This condition can have serious health implications and greatly increase LOS in the intensive care unit (ICU). To avoid such infections, patients should be appropriately managed based on clinical criteria for pulmonary toileting and for weaning patients from the ventilator if appropriate. In addition, self-extubation, which occurs when the patient rather than a clinician removes the ventilator tube, should be avoided because patients can injure themselves by removing the ventilator inappropriately. Appropriate management increases value in that the patient has a better quality of life and an earlier discharge from the ICU to the floor.

Various measures can be developed to assess ventilator safety, such as tracking the number of days a patient is on a ventilator, following appropriate weaning protocols, and noting rates of self-extubation. Improved outcomes are reductions in the number of days a patient is on a ventilator and in the number of patients who self-extubate. For the latter measure, for example, the numerator is the number of self-extubations over a given time period and the denominator is the number of people on ventilators over the same period. Another measure might be the number of ventilator-associated pneumonias over the number of days in the ICU. These measures are both quality and financial measures. Ventilator-associated pneumonias and injuries associated with self-extubation are preventable. Therefore the financial outlay associated with treatment of them is an indicator of waste.

care. Once an improvement has been proven effective, the new process is communicated throughout the organization.

This improvement methodology relies on common sense to evaluate outcomes and uses data as a basis of process improvement. Its cyclical and overlapping approach reinforces change and encourages communication among the various stakeholders involved in the process.

If improvement efforts are to be maintained, organizations need to use multidisciplinary input when determining evaluative measures and defining change. The traditional mortality and morbidity (M&M) review process involves physicians only and does not address areas of improvement that should be communicated across the health care organization. The quality management approach to problems stresses communication across the continuum and involves all relevant staff in developing and maintaining changed processes to improve outcomes (see Figure 4.2.). Because care is multidisciplinary, understanding gaps in care and suggesting improvements should be multidisciplinary as well.

EXAMPLE: TRANSPLANTS

The lucrative and highly specialized medical service of organ transplants offers a good example of the link between finance and quality. Transplants are among the most expensive *diagnosis-related groups (DRGs)*, which means that the organization gets paid more for transplants than other services. Therefore hospital administrators want to have transplant units.

However, care must be of the highest quality for a hospital to become credentialed in this financially rewarding service. The government requires mandatory reporting of quality indicators to monitor the safety of patients who need this highly specialized surgery. CMS compares the data for each transplant unit to the data for other transplant units. A unit has to earn the ranking of Center of Excellence and maintain excellent processes and outcomes. Data are reported on public Web sites so that patients can make informed choices about where to go for transplants. If a unit's

Using Guidelines to Improve Outcomes

In the current model of health care, the "product" being produced is treatment. This is readily understood when a patient with atherosclerosis requires an angioplasty but less easily defined when a patient has pneumonia. The product for a pneumonia patient is not one specific procedure but an entire treatment plan. As with other chronic diseases, such as heart failure, this treatment is based on evidence and managed with guidelines for appropriate and effective care.

FIGURE 4.2 Traditional and quality management modes of analysis

Morbidity and Mortality Review	Quality Management Analysis
• Deals only with case in question • Is reaction based • Is a closed-door review • Analyzes a specific incident • Reviews specific facts of a specific case • Uses improvement suggestions from peers • Teaches residents critical thinking • Involves an informal critique • Stresses individual competence	• Aggregates incidents or all similar cases • Examines commonalities or variations • Uses multidisciplinary analysis • Is proactive, not reactive • Focuses on process not outcome • Involves critical thinking for individuals • Shares information from teaching to hospital community • Moves from incident to hospital to system • Develops guidelines for best practice • Employs the PDCA cycle for continuous improvement • Establishes benchmarks from national or state data banks

data show poor outcomes, then CMS surveys the hospital, which is at risk of losing its license to perform transplants. Closing a unit due to poor quality costs the hospital enormous sums of money. Clearly, if performance is below standard, the organization will suffer financially.

Quality measures are defined to objectively assess the delivery of transplant care and to understand causes of complications and mortality. Some measures are established by CMS, such as tracking the number of grafts that fail. Other measures are established by each hospital. Quality management staff help to define the measure, collect the data, and interpret it for the organization. Quality staff meet with physicians and administrative leaders to discuss cases, do root cause analyses of problems, and participate in PDCA efforts for improvement. Measures help everyone involved identify trends. Monthly reports of quality variables improve communication and oversight.

DIAGNOSIS-RELATED GROUP (DRG) DRGs are the basis of the system that is used to classify patients and hospital resources in order to receive Medicaid and Medicare reimbursement (and usually other insurance reimbursement as well).

EXAMPLE: CARDIAC MORTALITY Another example of how measures can improve outcomes involves cardiac surgery. When one hospital determined to understand and reduce its mortality rate for cardiac surgery, it began an improvement initiative using the PDCA methodology. Data collection revealed that among the surgical patients who died, many had unplanned returns to the OR after surgery. When quality management staff analyzed the reason for the returns to the OR, it became apparent that there was an association between these returns and sternal wound infections. After drilling down further in the data, analysts concluded that bleeding was the primary cause of the infection. Due to these data and measures, physicians then modified their use of blood thinners for patients about to undergo surgery and used other prophylactic procedures to prevent bleeding. Bleeding was reduced; infection was reduced; unplanned returns to the OR were reduced; mortality was reduced. Everyone benefited. Patient outcomes were improved, data reported to the public were improved, and waste in the OR was reduced. Profit increased.

To maximize the effectiveness of this product line by disease or diagnosis, each treatment should be defined, along with who is responsible for delivering each step in the treatment plan and what outcome is anticipated from each intervention. The clinical pathway provides a detailed treatment plan by disease and signifies what to do each day for each patient.

Traditionally, physicians based patient care on their clinical experience. Today the focus is on the process of care and on incorporating into care defined measurements for treatment to ensure the patient's stability and recovery. Incorporating evidence-based medicine into care reduces variation; increasing standardization reduces costs. Evidence-based medicine should be considered a framework for treatment, with the clinician's experience providing the goals for the treatment plan. Because there are variations among patients, variances from the plan may occur, but they should be documented to either change the plan or explain the exception in the care.

Industry has successfully used performance improvement methodologies, including PDCA, to monitor production. When actions are the same and the unit of analysis and the outcome of production are well defined, variations or defects can be easily identified through inspections. When I had the responsibility of inspecting the repair of armored vehicles for the Israeli army, I was able to identify those vehicles that did not perform well when driven. A focused review showed that some mechanics were creative, which is to say that they allowed their own experience to override standard expectations. I realized then that even in the most routinized and well-defined processes there are variations in performance. Those variations are expensive because they necessitate rework and repair to bring the output, in this example a vehicle, to acceptable standards of performance. In health care too, maintaining the standards reduces the need for rework, that is, readmission to the hospital.

CMS encourages clinicians to follow a standardized treatment plan for chronic disease management by increasing reimbursement to those hospitals that document compliance with defined measures. These measures have been established because data show that when standardized treatment plans are followed, more patients have good outcomes than when these plans are not used. CMS has also defined specific exclusion criteria for its measures. For example, if a patient cannot be given a beta blocker as required by one measure, the physician is expected to document the reason for the variation in care. The documentation ensures that the lack of compliance with the standard is thoughtful and not a thoughtless omission.

An explicit treatment plan is also essential because patients often receive consults from many different disciplines. An appropriate plan fosters communication among all disciplines involved in the patient's care. An appropriate plan takes into consideration the patient's psychosocial issues that might have an impact on his or her responsiveness to treatment and to effective patient education. Taking the entire patient into account, rather than focusing solely on correcting a medical problem, produces a better relationship between caregiver and patient. Understanding the patient also leads to more effective and timely discharge planning and effective treatment throughout the continuum of care.

The clinical pathway based on guidelines is critical to prevention efforts because it embeds evidence-based medicine, the National Patient Safety Goals, and other measures of patient safety into the care plan. Despite all these advantages, clinical pathways are not universally implemented and in fact are often treated as an inconvenience that has little preventive power. Clinicians in many countries outside the United States, however, use clinical pathways without the complaint that documenting the daily treatment is useless paperwork.

Clinical pathways provide good value. Managers can plan for organizational efficiency because treatment is specified. Data for regulatory compliance are easily collected. Variance analysis explains the differences between the guidelines and the patient's ability to respond to the treatment plan. Retrospective analysis of variance data provides information that is useful for research and performance improvement initiatives. Clinical pathways can become a tool to measure waste.

Managing the Elderly Patient

As the patient population ages, elderly patients who have multiple health problems and chronic diseases often enter hospitals for an acute illness. Special skills and treatments are required to deal with this highly vulnerable, medically complex population. By tracking the care of the elderly patient in various settings, one hospital I worked with realized that there was a very poor transition from long-term care to acute care, that is, from a nursing facility to the hospital ED.

Quality management staff found that information about these patients was not being fully communicated. Many elderly patients were experiencing disorientation, but often the medical staff did not address the cognitive difficulty the patient was having; they were focused instead on dealing with the immediate medical crisis. It was not until a nursing home reported that its patients were returning from the acute care setting of the hospital in poorer condition than they had been when admitted that clinical and administrative leaders took notice and prioritized an inquiry into the cause. The nursing home reported that patients were being returned from the hospital with decubiti and increased psychosocial problems. When the nursing home threatened to send its patients elsewhere, the hospital leaders determined to address the problem and improve the process of care. The improvement initiative resulted in enhanced communication between the nursing home and the acute care facility and addressed specific problems of the elderly patient, such as medication reconciliation and appropriate nutrition.

Prevention is especially critical for the elderly patient. Many elderly patients are prescribed multiple medications and managing them is very complicated. It is easy to become confused and to take too much medication, the wrong medication, or not enough medication or to take it not at the right time or not in the way directed (for example, with food or without). When an elderly patient with complex medical problems is hospitalized for an acute episode of illness, new medications are often added to the existing medications and sometimes the hospital pharmacy dispenses a generic version of a patient's medication that may look different from what the patient is used to taking. At discharge, it has to be perfectly clear to the patient what to take: are the medications that the patient is discharged with consistent, appropriate, and understood by the patient?

To be sure that medication is appropriately managed the patient has to be educated. Unfortunately, there is no test to ensure that patients actually do understand or that they have been effectively taught. The government has stepped in to try to focus attention on this problem. The Joint Commission requires that compliance with the preventive measure, medication reconciliation, be documented in the patient's medical record. But it is easy to simply check that such education was offered; the checkmark does not reveal whether the information was understood or effective. Managing medication at discharge is more than a compliance issue. To increase prevention and to avoid having the patient return to the hospital for medical management, education should be more than compliance with a requirement. Education should be seen as preventive care for the patient and an effort to improve organizational efficiency and eliminate waste for the health care institution.

End-of Life Issues   Data have had an important impact on changing the way hospitals care for patients at the end of life. I saw the influence of data on care decisions firsthand when the North Shore-LIJ Health System introduced the APACHE database into its ICUs. APACHE (an acronym for Acute Physiology and Chronic Health Evaluation) is a predictive tool that defines the population in an ICU in terms of severity of illness and the patients' need for services. Information about the severity of patient illness assists in the efficient prioritization of resources. The APACHE database is also a preventive tool, because when clinicians can define whether patients can benefit from interventions or not, unnecessary procedures and pain are avoided.

In our case APACHE data highlighted the fact that many of the patients in the ICUs were very ill and at the end of life. They had little need for highly technical or specialized services; they needed palliative care. This information about how the ICUs were being used provoked important questions about what services should be provided for the very sick. To what extent should invasive procedures be performed on the terminally ill? What is the role of comfort care and of do not resuscitate and do not intubate (DNR and DNI) orders at the end of life? Should heroic measures be taken to prolong life? Who should decide?

Often it is difficult to distinguish between clinical and ethical issues, especially because ethical questions arise in the hospital setting and involve clinicians. When the APACHE data alerted the clinicians in our health system that ICU care might be overutilized and inappropriately utilized, staff worked to establish new policies. A multidisciplinary task force formulated criteria for appropriate admittance and discharge to the unit and formulated other policies that took into account the clinician, the patient, and the patient's family. The effort to develop meaningful policies for the end-of-life patient increased communication among all the people involved in the patient's care. The data pointed out trends that led to better defined processes. Clinicians were forced to think about care in a new way. Before the data analysis, everyone who was gravely ill had ended up in an ICU, regardless of services required.

By reducing waste in the ICUs and by better managing the care of end-of-life patients, the health care system enhanced the value of these units. At the same time, end-of-life patients received excellent and appropriate care, such as hospice care. Guidelines were developed for effective and humane management of their care. It is far less expensive for a health care organization to provide end-of-life patients with dignified and compassionate care than it is to impose inappropriate tests and procedures on these patients. The ratio of staff to patient is low; expensive services are not required. Without the support of data, however, it is difficult to reach this level of understanding of appropriateness of care.

Dartmouth Atlas of Health Care Study   A study reported in *The Dartmouth Atlas of Health Care 2008* used Medicare data from seventy-seven health systems and about five million patients with chronic diseases around the United States to examine end-of-life care. The results of this data analysis brought the nation's attention to the great variability in the amount and type of health care services provided by hospitals to terminal patients. The research showed that these services depended on the resources available at particular hospitals and not on standards rooted in evidence-based medicine. Researchers collected information about how many days each patient spent in the ICU, how many days the patient spent in the hospital, the number of physician visits the patient had during his or her stay, and the number of patients who saw more than ten physicians during their final six months of life.

The researchers concluded that receiving more care (days in an ICU and physician visits) did not extend life expectancy. In other words, quality was not correlated with utilization. Patients were using expensive resources without gaining any real benefit.

The study helped to raise consciousness about why patients use certain resources and what criteria should be applied to their use. The recognition of overtreatment and of variation in care has led to a movement to establish palliative care units and hospice care. Patients at the end of life benefit from hospice care, not from excessive, expensive, painful, and unnecessary interventions. APACHE data have helped organizations distinguish between those patients who can use ICU resources and those who can be better treated with another level of care. Until large databases accurately reflected care, this type of resource evaluation was impossible. The data established that for end-of-life patients there was no return on investment. There was no value. However, this recognition led to a reduction in patients' stay in the ICU and the development of appropriate criteria for admission to the ICU and other levels of care.

SUMMARY

In order to best understand the relationship among processes, outcomes, and costs, strategies such as the following are useful

- Monitor never events

- Use quality data in purchasing decisions

- Define waste reduction as an indicator of efficiency

- Document quality indicators for increased reimbursement and lower insurance expenses

- Implement and monitor improvements with the PDCA process

- Establish criteria for end-of-life care

KEY TERMS

APACHE   PDCA
end-of-life care   waste
never events

THINGS TO THINK ABOUT

Imagine that you are in charge of the ICU at your hospital. How will you ensure that the patients are appropriate, that the patients receive excellent care, and that ICU resources are being used appropriately?

1. What criteria would you use to evaluate the appropriateness of the patient population?

2. What kinds of data would you collect to argue that the resources of the unit are being used efficiently?

3. What criteria and what data would you use to evaluate the quality of care patients receive on the unit?

4. What information would you present to the CFO to prove that the unit was efficient?

PART

2

GETTING DOWN
TO BUSINESS

CHAPTER

5

THE VALUE OF PREVENTION

LEARNING OBJECTIVES

- Discuss various government attempts at promoting prevention
- Discuss barriers to health care organizations' support of prevention strategies
- Explain the role of data, databases, and measurements in improving outcomes
- Discuss issues of prevention in the ambulatory setting
- Explain the value of using the FMEA methodology to promote prevention

There is no doubt that prevention saves lives and improves the management of chronic illness; for this reason, prevention will be a major focus of health care activities in the future. Preventing illness is better for patients and much more economical for health care organizations than treating disease during acute phases of illness. As the population ages, people are living longer with (often multiple) chronic diseases. Problems such as diabetes, cardiovascular diseases, and chronic respiratory diseases affect millions of people and overtax our health care systems. These diseases also respond to prevention efforts and are associated with preventable risk factors. Smoking, nutrition, exercise, and proper management of medication and other lifestyle factors have an impact on these diseases, and physicians are beginning to include education and information about these topics in routine patient visits. Chronic diseases must be well managed or, preferably, prevented so that they do not generate health care costs that will seriously deplete our already burdened health care system.

THE PROMOTION OF PREVENTION

For many years health organizations such as the American Heart Association have been stressing the importance of prevention in maintaining health. Many people have taken seriously their doctors' recommendations to eat a healthier diet, get regular exercise, stop smoking, and reduce alcohol intake, and these preventive steps, along with medical interventions, have reduced the death rates from cardiovascular disease over the past few decades.

There is even a national task force on prevention, called the U.S. Preventive Services Task Force, sponsored by the Agency for Healthcare Research and Quality (AHRQ), which enlists experts to evaluate the effectiveness of various preventive services, such as screening and medications. The task force makes recommendations in numerous clinical categories and now recommends screening older adults (over age sixty-five) for chronic diseases because data show that screening has proved effective. For example, data from multiple trials reveal that screening for and treating hypertension reduces mortality. Screening for breast, cervical, and colorectal cancers has also been shown to reduce mortality. Vaccines against flu and pneumonia are recommended for people over age sixty because data show that they reduce the number of illnesses and hospitalizations as well as lowering mortality.

AHRQ has also instituted a national program, called Put Prevention Into Practice, to increase preventive services such as immunizations, screening tests, and information given to patients. The agency has developed preventive quality indicators that measure which conditions that have resulted in patient hospitalizations might have been avoided through adequate preventive care in the outpatient environment.

Other initiatives, such as Healthy People 2010, a federal program built on earlier efforts to promote health by preventing disease, have established national objectives for health care. The Healthy People 2010 program identifies preventable threats to health and defines goals to reduce these threats. Program objectives are monitored through health indicator data collected from various governmental agencies.

The World Health Organization has said that every health care interaction should be an opportunity to provide prevention education and support. Education about reducing risks for illness can significantly reduce the health care cost burden.

Insurance companies and health maintenance organizations (HMOs) want to reduce hospital and medical expenses by focusing on prevention and rewarding organizations and physicians who demonstrate compliance with preventive measures. Obviously, it is to their advantage; without the extreme resource consumption of hospitalizations, expenses would be lowered. The idea behind managed care was to prevent hospitalization through appropriate management in the physician's office and through prevention. The concept was good, but implementation was very difficult. Managed care became a utilization review tool, and unfortunately, the focus became the criteria for denial of payment for hospital services rather than clinical preventive measures.

It is indisputable that prevention provides good value—for the patient, who remains in better health, and for the health care industry, which avoids extraordinary and unnecessary expenses. Win win. One would think there would be a great deal of support for preventive measures. But as you will see, introducing prevention into health care organizations involves very complex issues and exposes interesting conflicts of interest.

THE PROBLEMS WITH PREVENTION

With so much information about the value of prevention, it is curious that health care organizations do not aggressively support the effort of promoting prevention. One primary issue is that clinicians are not adequately trained in prevention. On the contrary, hospitals and physicians are focused on treating disease and reacting to emergencies. The entire social structure of the hospital is built around identifying and curing illness—not preventing it. In other words, hospitals react. Prevention is not reacting. Prevention involves anticipating a possible outcome and taking steps to control the environment to avoid a poor outcome and also to examine risk factors and then attempt to eliminate them. The hospital environment is not conducive to such proactive anticipation.

The economic model of medicine is especially unfriendly to introducing prevention efforts and supporting the management of chronic conditions. Often there is little or no reimbursement for preventive services. Under our current system, physicians get paid for managing illness—not wellness. Hospitals and physicians do not get paid if patients are healthy. Also, hospitals are engaged in promoting efficiency rather than quality. However, this idea is economically shortsighted; the hospital may reap some immediate financial benefits by a quick turnover in the operating room (OR), a high volume of expensive radio-logical tests, and a short length of stay (LOS), but in the long run it will lose money if the quality of care is poor. Poor management of illness and chronic disease results in low reimbursements. Ideally, efficiency should be defined as a subset of quality. Poor quality is not efficient. Efficiency does not necessarily promote quality. Moreover, prevention efforts are successful for outpatient clinics, but for hospitals they are not a source of income as are inpatient services. Hospital administrators often consider outpatient services to be an economic burden or a social service to the community.

The problems involved in promoting prevention seem intractable. The hospital cannot be involved with patients postdischarge. No one comes into the patients' homes to ensure that they are taking their medications properly and complying with their diet and exercise regimens. Busy physicians working in hospitals are responsible for taking care of hospitalized patients. Furthermore, attending physicians do not get paid to search for their patients' primary care doctors in the community and discussing preventive follow-up care with them. For hospital doctors, there is no financial incentive associated with prevention. Their work and their income depend on the treatment of disease.

A paradigm shift is essential if we are to change the focus of health care management, moving from a reactive culture to a culture that focuses on prevention and maintenance, and from stressing only efficiency to stressing quality. Government is attempting to influence this shift by rewarding organizations financially for documenting compliance with preventive measures and penalizing hospitals financially if there is no compliance. However, even with governmental pressure, there are enormous challenges in changing the health care culture, a culture that has shaped physicians' behavior and belief systems for years and is rooted in the socialization process of medical schools and of residency and fellowship programs that stress having autonomy, enjoying professional privacy, reacting to problems, and being the sole authority in judging excellent care.

THE PATIENT'S ROLE

Prevention and disease management depend primarily on patient behavior. However, even when programs are effective and physicians and patients believe in the value of prevention, subtle social forces reduce people's commitment to improving patient safety. Even well-motivated patients who want to participate in their own care and believe in establishing a patient-focused environment have trouble following preventive instructions. Everyone knows that smoking is not good for one's health, yet people continue to smoke. We all know that exercise has many health benefits, yet most of us do not exercise adequately. The diet industry is making zillions of dollars because even though people want to be slim, they also want to eat what they want to eat.

Long-term health gains are clearly less compelling than immediate gratification. Prevention is a long-term enterprise.

To best manage their conditions, patients with chronic diseases have to be willing to follow medical advice about medication, exercise, diet, follow-up visits to the doctor, and immunizations. With the best of intentions, it is difficult for physicians to continuously monitor their patients' behavior once those patients are out of the hospital setting. In a hospital the patient is acted upon: medicine is delivered, administered, and monitored; procedures are performed; and so forth. Once the patient is discharged from the hospital and in the home environment, taking medication is a personal choice. There is no way for the health care professional to maintain vigilance over the patient's behavior once the person is outside the highly controlled universe of the hospital. If a patient has diabetes and is not supposed to eat sweets but indulges in sweet desserts anyway, what can a physician do? Physicians cannot force people to comply with standards of care. They can provide education to the best of their ability, but after that it is up to the patient.

To attempt to overcome these multiple barriers to prevention, the government has taken action to promote measures and develop methods to encourage prevention.

PREVENTION MEASURES

The Centers for Medicare and Medicaid Services (CMS) is attempting to change existing medical culture by financially rewarding hospitals that comply with evidence-based measures of prevention in their delivery of care. Objective data are the weapons of choice for making needed changes in practice and encouraging clinicians and administrators to rethink their existing modes of behavior. The pressure to not be seen as below average is encouraging change.

The government is focusing on the management of chronic diseases in particular because these high-volume conditions would have an enormous and beneficial financial and clinical impact if properly managed. Before CMS required the process variables associated with pneumonia to be measured, the only measures hospitals collected for this illness were the volume of pneumonia patients, LOS, and case mix index—all financial indicators. Mortality (not risk adjusted) was also collected but only for medical education through discussion in mortality and morbidity (M&M) case conferences. But because specific process measures, such as the timing of antibiotic delivery and appropriate discharge, are now required, care has improved. The intent of collecting process variables is to reduce variation in care as much as possible. Variation in the practice of managing disease is very costly and does not necessarily result in good outcomes.

CMS expects documentation of a timely and accurate diagnosis and timely and appropriate treatment. The requirement to comply with such process measures improves patient outcomes and ensures that resources are used appropriately and interventions quickly provided. Everyone benefits. Physician behavior is modified; the chief financial officer (CFO) pays attention; and leadership sets new expectations for the hospital, changing the focus to the quality of care delivered in addition to the volume of patients admitted with complex diagnosis-related group (DRG) classifications and the reduction of LOS. Indicators, such as timely antibiotic administration for pneumonia, incorporate an efficiency measure into a clinical quality measure.

National benchmarks for good care, based on evidence and data, have been developed for pneumonia and other conditions. Before being exposed to the influence of publicly reported data, individual physicians diagnosed and treated pneumonia patients idiosyncratically, individually, and subjectively; treatment varied based on each physician's experience, attendance at continuing education programs, and diligence in keeping up with research reported in the literature. Now physicians are expected to diagnose pneumonia based on evidence that may not be in line with their experience.

Expert physicians define these quality variables, not insurers. These measures have been adopted because research shows that patient outcomes improve when physicians comply with the measures. If standardized care is not appropriate for certain patients, then these exceptions to the standard need to be documented in the medical record for compliance. When a physician compares the exception to the norm and asks why a particular patient is inappropriate for standard treatment, the focus is on the patient's condition. Documentation ensures that if a pneumonia patient is not given the standard antibiotic, it is due to a deliberate and conscious decision rather than to poor communication, lost reports, poor memory, or incompetence. For many caregivers, documenting compliance with the required indicators is a nuisance. Often physicians do not take seriously the documenting of preventive safety measures. Although CMS and other governmental agencies can attempt to influence behavior, they can only do so much. For the measures to be effective, clinicians must buy into the understanding that using these measures is to the patient's and the organization's and their own advantage and that these measures promote improved outcomes.

REGULATORY GROUPS' ROLE IN PREVENTION

Health care regulatory agencies, such as the Joint Commission, approach prevention by focusing on patient safety and error reduction. In addition to requiring that health care organizations comply with preventive health care measurements, they also require documentation about processes that have been developed to prevent errors. If a hospital has an incident that has an impact on patient safety, surveyors from agencies such as the Joint Commission expect to find that a root cause analysis has been performed and that corrective actions have been developed. If an unexpected outcome occurs, such as mortality, then the Joint Commission investigates whether procedures were in place that might have avoided the poor outcome, whether those procedures were followed, and if not, why not and what is being done to correct the procedures. The goal is always to promote a commitment to safer, patient-centered care and to prevent preventable errors.

The Joint Commission's tracer methodology (also discussed in Chapters Two and Eight) was developed to help surveyors track the details of a patient's episode of hospitalization. The surveyors inquire into all the processes involved during the hospitalization and look to see not only whether the correct steps were followed along the way but also whether communication was effective, whether appropriate information was transferred, and whether staff were focused on the patient's care.

The Joint Commission's survey process is dynamic. The surveyors question whomever they wish to in the hospital, at every level of care, and not just a few individuals chosen in advance. They ask staff why an event took place and what staff members know about proper procedure. Everyone is supposed to be involved in the safety efforts. They check the medical record to make sure it is complete, that the lab results have been entered, and that orders were fulfilled in a timely way. They review the clinical and organization response to the lab tests through progress notes. Then they review the way the pharmacy prepared the patient's medication, for example, an antibiotic for pneumonia, and whether an appropriate patient profile detailing allergies and other medications that might cause a reaction was in place prior to ordering the antibiotic.

The pharmacy would also be reviewed to see whether the antibiotic was appropriately labeled, dispensed in a timely way, and delivered to the unit. Then the nurses' behavior would be traced to determine whether the antibiotic was administered correctly, on time, and in the right way. In short, the tracer methodology is a highly detailed examination of the process of care designed to ascertain whether organizations are taking steps to protect the patient from harm and to prevent errors caused by gaps in the process of care. By making the tracer central to the accreditation process, the Joint Commission is forcing health care organizations to focus attention on any breakdowns in the efficient and effective flow of care. However, such efforts are limited because maintaining readiness is not a continuing process, and many administrators still see these efforts by regulators as an expense rather than as a motivator for change.

DATA'S ROLE IN PROMOTING PREVENTION

The use of data to evaluate hospital care by governmental agencies is contributing to changing the traditional culture in which individual physicians treat individual patients according to their own training and experience and answer to no one other than perhaps during M&M case conferences if there is a problem in the delivery of care. Clinicians, administrators, and staff are gaining an increased understanding of the variables that can be used to define processes, outcomes, and quality care. Even if the data are not methodologically "clean," the national movement to report and compare hospital care has influenced payments, processes, and public relations. Data have also influenced physician behavior.

By risk adjusting data about large patient populations and by developing appropriate measures for care, agencies and researchers are developing new models for treating diseases for entire populations rather than only individual patients. Through the use of large databases and statistical analyses, expectations about outcomes, such as mortality rates or readmissions, can be objectively defined.

Data that turn into valuable information for the physician have the potential to save lives. Gathering data and evaluating care in an objective way is slowly changing the traditional culture of health care. Individual subjectivity, the so-called art of medicine, is being replaced by norms, variables, evidence-based measures, and statistical analyses of aggregated data. By grouping patients into populations and analyzing process and outcome variables in databases, researchers provide caregivers with information about common characteristics and a way to understand and refine processes for disease management. For example, analyzing why one surgical patient had to be readmitted to the OR provides less information than analyzing why a group of such patients had to be readmitted. Common clinical characteristics can be analyzed, as can specific medical interventions; these variables can be coupled with demographic information and trended to understand the readmittances. Aggregated data allow caregivers to find the common thread. By focusing on the expected outcome, caregivers can investigate variation from the standard. Providing quality services results in money saved for the hospital.

HealthGrades, an organization that uses data to rank the quality of care in hospitals (and by physician) across the nation, with data that are risk-adjusted for valid comparisons, is influencing the delivery of care by publicly reporting comparative ranking of outcomes. Poor rankings might influence value by lowering a hospital's patient census, increasing its malpractice insurance costs, and reducing reimbursements. Bad report cards diminish value.

When HealthGrades reported that mortality was higher than the national average for heart failure patients treated at one of the hospitals in the multihospital health care system where I work, the leadership asked me to investigate the problem. By examining administrative data, my research team was able to identify secondary diagnoses associated with heart failure mortality. Ventilator-associated infections, urinary tract infections (UTIs), and decubiti (all preventable) were found to be associated with heart failure mortality. These kinds of connections and analyses are possible only with large databases. The findings from large databases suggest treatment options and performance improvement targets that might otherwise be obscured.

Data help to explain complications. For example, if a patient expires with a diagnosis of sepsis, an interesting and important question to investigate is why this patient died and other similar patients did not. More generally, the question to ask is, What is the relationship between infection and mortality? Is it a random event or part of a process that can be improved? After the health care organization analyzes how different variables interact with mortality, policies can be developed. If processes are developed to focus on lowering infection, mortality may decrease. Infection rates relate to process variables (what was done to the patient) and mortality to outcomes (what happened to the patient). By matching process and outcome variables and analyzing the data statistically, researchers can retrieve important information.

Other questions that can be asked are, What contributes to increased infection rates? And what guidelines can be developed to reduce an infection rate? Although physicians have known for decades that infection influences mortality, the large databases now available that show correlations are more effective in forcing changed policies. The information is not new, but the sheer size of the data set compels new policies. For example, data show that wound infections are quite common after surgery; they are also expensive to treat. Data also show that administering a prophylactic antibiotic can reduce infection, lower mortality, and save money by reducing unintended expenses, such as readmission to the hospital. Now physicians are more likely to administer prophylactic antibiotics not so much because of evidence but due to pressure from administrators to comply in order that the hospital not be viewed as a "poor performer."

When hospitals focus on data, prevention efforts increase. When report cards compare mortality rankings, steps are taken to reduce mortality. When data show that stroke patients who receive clot-dissolving medication (tissue plasminogen activator, or t-PA) quickly have a better outcome than those who do not receive timely medication, the management of the stroke patient changes. Data are driving the promotion of guidelines that clinicians can use for their own benefit and that of their patients.

Through data, organizations gain knowledge, and knowledge can improve prevention efforts. For example, when quality management staff at the North Shore—LIJ Health System tracked data on complications following bariatric surgery, it became apparent that not all physicians were equally competent to perform this complicated surgery. Data showed that clinicians with very little experience had a much higher complication rate than more experienced physicians did. This type of information is available only when data are analyzed in the aggregate rather than for one physician at a time. Based on this information, new protocols for credentialing were developed to help improve physician competence and new protocols were developed for post-surgical support. Mortality decreased; patients were safer; complications were prevented; expenses decreased.

Primary data, gathered from electronic medical records (EMRs), will become increasingly available for data analysis. Data will be garnered easily from the EMRs and be more complete and accurate than data extracted from individual progress notes of individual medical records. Databases that have traditionally been used for reimbursement will be used to understand outcomes. Primary data will be submitted to insurance companies and will begin to drive changed practices.

Happily, many physicians are beginning to understand the value of analyzing large populations and using measures to evaluate care. This change in attitude, from subjective to objective, has enabled health care professionals to ask new questions. For example, if 99 percent of patients have no complications from some treatment or procedure, but 1 percent die, is that figure tolerable and expected, or should that 1 percent (which may in fact be equal to large numbers of people) be investigated in order to identify improvements in care? Every fraction of a percentage point reflects improved care. What happened to the 1 percent who died? Are there noticeable trends that can be identified and improved? If mortality is compared across organizations, do some organizations do better than others? Clinicians can ask what processes made the results different.

EXAMPLE: DVTs

Data show that blood clots (deep vein thromboses, or DVTs) frequently occur in patients who have had orthopedic surgery. This dangerous situation is preventable. Once measures identify a patient population where targeted prevention efforts would make an impact, therapeutic interventions can be developed.

Data showed my hospital system that orthopedic patients, who spend many hours immobilized both in the OR and in postsurgical care, were most susceptible to getting DVTs. A multidisciplinary task force was convened to analyze the causes of the DVTs and to make recommendations for improvements. Because there were many suspected causes, many solutions were implemented. For example, patients were positioned differently in the OR and every attempt was made to shorten the time spent in the OR. Also, heparin, a blood-thinning medication, was given to orthopedic patients prophylactically before surgery, to reduce the possibility of a clot forming, and special stockings designed to reduce clots were given to patients after surgery. These interventions made a difference. DVTs were dramatically reduced for orthopedic patients. When problems are analyzed and improvements implemented, patients have better outcomes.

EXAMPLE: STROKE PATIENTS AND ASPIRATION PNEUMONIA

When our health system determined to reduce the mortality rate of stroke patients, the first step was to attempt to understand the cause of the mortality. After a careful review of the patients who died, two common factors were revealed: most stroke patients who died were elderly, and many had a secondary diagnosis of aspiration pneumonia. Without analysis of aggregated data, we would not have been aware of these variables.

Aspiration pneumonia is a serious lung infection usually caused by breathing in foreign material, such as food or vomit. Patients who have trouble swallowing because they are comatose or only semiconscious or have a problem with their gag reflex are prone to this condition. Stroke patients are particularly vulnerable.

Once this association was identified, we took steps to introduce swallowing therapy for stroke patients. Speech and swallowing consultations helped to train stroke patients in ways to swallow their food. Aspiration pneumonia decreased. Mortality decreased. Information, analysis, and improvements saved lives.

MANAGEMENT OF CHRONIC CONDITIONS

When report cards publicly expose hospitals with poor outcomes, such as high rates of mortality or infection, health care institutions are spurred to invest in reducing rates of mortality and infection and in chronic disease management. For example, when data reveal that heart failure patients who die tend to be those who require readmission to the hospital, several lines of investigation seem worth examining to discover the cause of those readmissions. Patients generally come to the hospital because they are experiencing acute problems. Because heart failure is a chronic disease that responds to management, investigation should be conducted to learn what led to the acute episodes. Several reasons are possible: the patient had an idiosyncratic episode; the original care in the hospital was not adequate to control the disease; the discharge instructions were incomplete or poorly understood; the follow-up care instructions were not followed or were inadequate.

Once an organization determines to investigate a high mortality rate and then takes steps to reduce that rate through proactive prevention, it might be useful to predict which patients are most vulnerable. To make such a prediction, hospitals require detailed risk assessment tools. But before these tools can be developed, data are needed about the specific patient population. Without a well-defined numerator and denominator, which is to say, without good measures describing a particular population, it is very difficult to develop preventive methods. For example, if the organization prioritizes the prevention of nosocomial pneumonia in the ICU or the prevention of postoperative blood clots, it needs information about those patients who suffer from these problems in order to design the prevention. Data may help to reveal why the adverse event occurs and then improvements can be implemented to prevent it.

Measures pinpoint a problem and identify a population. Once an intervention is developed, measures should be defined to assess whether the intervention was effective, that is, if the desired outcome was attained. Are there, for example, fewer blood clots occurring postsurgery for the orthopedic patient population? The organization can document that the anticlotting medication was in fact administered and can track outcomes of patients to confirm that the medication made a difference to postoperative complications. Physicians can get on board with these measures because they can see the value. The organization can get behind these measures as well because complications cost the organization in terms of LOS and resource consumption.

The more health care organizations measure and the more they analyze the delivery of care, the more they can increase prevention by lowering maloccurrences. Most measures are actually preventive, especially those required by the government. For example, before a procedure is performed, the Joint Commission and CMS require medical clearance from the physician that the patient is appropriate for the procedure. The intent of this requirement—which has to be documented and measured for reporting—is to reduce complications. A thorough preoperative history and physical identifies any potential problems in advance of the procedure and decreases the chances for complications and mortality.

Another measure of prevention, one that is both clinical and organizational, involves the emergency department (ED). Measures can be developed to track which patients are admitted and which are not and whether patients who are admitted, treated, and released return and are readmitted. The group of readmitted patients can then be analyzed to assess whether the original care was inadequate or whether the patients have common characteristics or a common diagnosis. Perhaps there is another kind of flaw in the process, a procedure that should be performed but is not being performed. In other words, measures that track the rate of readmissions can be used to define a problem area. Root cause analysis of the set of patients being targeted can specify whether the issue is competency or something else. Having that information can lead to improvements, which in turn function as prevention for future patients.

Other measures of prevention mitigate problems before they become serious medical conditions. For example, research shows that women who have gestational diabetes have a higher risk for developing type 2 diabetes later in life than women who do not have gestational diabetes. These women often do not have symptoms associated with diabetes and therefore remain undiagnosed and untreated. Once this problem was recognized in the North Shore-LIJ

Health System, clinicians improved the diabetes screening of postpartum patients. Those patients with gestational diabetes were recommended for rescreening six weeks after delivery. They were also educated about diet and, if necessary, were referred to endocrinologists for follow-up treatment.

The care of diabetic patients generally was also the focus of a performance improvement effort in our health system. Guidelines exist for treating diabetic patients. For example, a blood test called a hemoglobin A1c (HbA1c) test, should be performed every three months to assess sugar levels. Blood pressure and cholesterol should be monitored as well. People with diabetes are vulnerable to foot injuries and eye problems and should have regular checkups with appropriate professionals. To ensure that physicians were following these guidelines, we reviewed a random sample of patient charts for compliance with the preventive indicators. Results of the review showed that every patient reviewed had four or more clinic visits during the year studied. They all had their HbA1c levels checked. Slightly more than half the patients had their blood pressure controlled. Less than 70 percent had had a retinal exam. Only 60 percent had documented patient education about their diabetes treatments. Once these data were collected and reported, physicians could target areas for improvements. Without the aggregated data analysis, these trends would not have been noted.

PREVENTION IN AMBULATORY CARE

The management of chronic diseases is most effectively accomplished in the ambulatory care setting. Ideally, this care will be effective enough to avoid acute episodes and hospitalizations. To promote prevention and improve care in the ambulatory settings associated with our health care system, I formed a special subcommittee of the quality committee of the board of trustees, whose responsibility was to oversee ambulatory services. The committee included clinicians, administrators, and quality management professionals, and the members met monthly to review indicators specific to the ambulatory setting.

The reason for trustee involvement was to increase accountability and to shift the focus of medical quality management from the hospital to the community, reinforce the continuum of care postdischarge, and close the loop of care. Without governance involvement, this shift will not occur because the reality of care delivery is that different physicians have patients being treated at different levels of care, and communication between community physicians and inpatient physicians is very poor. In fact, one reason for hospitals' low identification of postoperative wound infections is underreporting. Patients with such infections are often treated in the physician's office, and the hospital is not informed that a problem has occurred. Without such information, the hospital cannot assess the risks to patient safety or improve care.

FIGURE 5.1 *Ambulatory services table of measures*

EXAMPLE	PRIOR 12-MONTH AVERAGE	PRIOR 3-MONTH AVERAGE	CURRENT MONTH		
Operational Indicators					
examples					
Appointment Compliance Rate					
No Show Rate					
Clinical Indicators					
examples					
Compliance Rate for Pap Smear					
Compliance Rate for Mammography					

Measures for performance in the ambulatory clinics in our system were defined and monitored over time. Figure 5.1 shows examples of both operational and clinical indicators defined by the team. These and other measures were tracked over time and compared with the previous year's results. The lay members of the board's quality committee became familiar with performance goals and variations from the standards established through the consensus of experts. They held the community physicians accountable for the care those physicians gave.

The government appreciates the problems specific to the ambulatory setting and is trying to address the issue of prevention in that setting by developing programs, measures, and incentives to promote compliance. Programs such as Healthy People 2010 incorporate the use of preventive measures, but the obstacles to compliance are enormous.

Clinic patients in our system are often transient and there is often no continuum of care and no consistent relationship between patient and physician. Therefore preventive efforts in the clinic situation can be difficult. If, for example, a woman has a mammogram and requires follow-up treatment, there is no structure to ensure that she gets the follow-up or that the doctor she chooses to see has appropriate information and radiology results. If a person should get screened for breast cancer or cervical cancer or get a flu shot or the pneumonia vaccine, he or she makes the choice whether or not to take this preventive step.

Community doctors are trying to develop programs to encourage prevention among the outpatient community. There are health fairs, community screening opportunities, and support groups for people with specific diseases. However, these efforts do not yield great results. Well people often avoid interacting with the medical community, and they do not take advantage of outpatient prevention opportunities. When they need a doctor, they simply go to the ED.

The medical community is now focusing attention on the large number of people who use the ED as a proxy for a primary care physician. These people, especially those who do not have a relationship with a physician, come to the hospital in acute distress. For example, in winter they may have pneumonia and often they are elderly. As inpatients they have an extended LOS, for which the reimbursement is low. If these patients had been immunized and cared for in the outpatient setting, their rate of illness and of hospitalization might go down. Everyone would benefit.

Measures have been useful in highlighting problem areas in the ambulatory setting. For example, appointments are preventive, and patient attendance is relatively easy to measure. If a patient has missed an appointment, it is easily documented. Individuals who do not follow up with their physician or avoid coming to the office for monitoring have poorer outcomes than those patients do who comply with their physician's recommendations for office visits. The measure of attendance is also an indicator of efficiency, because missed appointments interrupt the clinics' daily workflow. To try to improve patient safety, the Joint Commission requires for accreditation that ambulatory centers and clinics pursue missing patients with follow-up phone calls and letters. However, people cannot be forced or compelled to come to a physician's office, and often their health suffers as a result.

Another challenge related to caring for the community outside the hospital involves maintaining communication along the continuum of care. For example, after an episode of hospitalization it is crucial that clinical information documenting the patient's treatment be transferred to the patient's physician. The patient's physician should get a copy of the discharge instructions as well so that he or she can supervise follow-up care.

However, health care organizations often have no process in place to transfer such information and no one is made accountable for this transfer. Hospital physicians cannot spend time tracking down the physicians of individual patients and making sure files are complete, copied, and transferred. Other clinical staff are also hard-pressed to fulfill their responsibilities during their shifts. Nonetheless, to maintain the continuum of care, and to prevent rehospitalizations, these kinds of problems need to be resolved.

It is also important to maintain lines of communication as patients move between levels of care, such as from the hospital into long-term care or between the nursing home and the ED. Ideally, the treatment plan should move along with the patient.

EXAMPLE: PROMOTING PREVENTION IN THE AMBULATORY SETTING

At one of the clinics associated with a community hospital in the North Shore-LIJ Health System, the staff and physicians realized that patients were missing a large number of appointments. They also understood that significant cultural, linguistic, and social barriers needed to be overcome before the people in the community effectively used the clinic for prevention. Leaders had to think outside the traditional box to develop processes that would bring reluctant patients into care and, once they were there, be responsive enough to their needs to keep them returning for follow-up and preventive care.

A set of measurements was developed that would capture both administrative data, such as volume and appointment compliance, and clinical data on preventive health care indicators, such as immunization of two-year-olds, Pap tests, and mammograms. The staff also collected demographic data and found that almost 80 percent of the patients in the clinic's community were Spanish speaking. The clinic leaders responded to this information by increasing the Spanish-speaking staff to almost 55 percent of the total staff. However, there were many other problems to address. A large percentage of the community residents were uninsured, and many were undocumented. They were unfamiliar with and suspicious of institutional settings. Yet they had many health problems that needed to be addressed.

Efforts have been made to improve the community's understanding of the health care services available to them and to encourage prevention. For example, the women's health program offers routine Pap smears and mammograms. To make sure that patients follow up if necessary, the nurses at the clinic developed a Pap educational form in Spanish and English that explains that the patient can

EXAMPLE: CARE FOR CHILDREN IN THE AMBULATORY SETTING

In order to provide access to care in underserved and high-risk communities throughout our region, we determined to bring medical services directly into the community. System leaders supported the creation of a pediatric mobile health center, housed in a recreational vehicle outfitted with three exam rooms, a nursing station, and a registration area. The van is staffed by a physician, nurse practitioner, medical assistant, social worker, and registrar. The staff are multilingual to better serve the patient population, and speak Spanish, Cantonese, and Hebrew in addition to English.

The van targets communities where a needs assessment has found the highest number of poor children and the lowest number of pediatric primary care providers.

expect to receive a letter if a follow-up appointment is required. The staff explain that the letter will be sent by both registered and regular mail. This explanation is important; staff are sensitive to the patients' fears about getting official mail relating to their immigration status. If an abnormal Pap test requires a colposcopic exam, one-to-one education is given to explain to the patient what to expect and how to schedule an appointment. Patients always have access to the staff, and they frequently make use of this option.

Childhood immunization is another example of the clinic's preventive health focus. In order to ensure that all children were fully immunized by two years of age, the charts of children under two are reviewed for immunization status at every visit. Now the clinic has 100 percent compliance with immunization requirements for two-year-olds.

All the staff's efforts to improve preventive care paid off. Improvement was seen on every measure. Appointment compliance went up 10 percent in a year, and the entire pediatric population was insured through Child Health Plus. Pregnancy tests were available daily, and if a test was positive, a resident immediately took a history and screened the patient. When appropriate, social services would be enlisted to provide the expectant mother with prenatal information and other support services.

Developing this program has required time and attention of a kind that is difficult to implement. However, the caring, innovative program and the significant improvement in health status for the community have made it worth the effort. With the commitment of clinic leaders to meet the challenges of the community through empowering the frontline staff to analyze, identify, and implement improvements, patients are now able to negotiate past multiple barriers to access compassionate, quality health care.

The goal is to improve access by delivering care directly to the community and to target chronic diseases such as tuberculosis, diabetes, asthma, and hypertension for intervention and education. In addition, the van provides well-child exams, immunizations, health screening (vision and hearing), and lead and cholesterol screening. Children who are sick are seen regardless of their insurance status. Parents are educated about health promotion and disease prevention, especially for asthma because of its prevalence among indigent children. When referrals are necessary, a pediatric physician associated with the hospital provides continuity of care.

In its first year of operation, the van saw an increase in revisits. Out of almost 3,000 primary care visits, 2,316 were revisits. The revisit indicates that the community has come to accept and trust the program. This innovative approach to preventive health for children has been an unqualified success.

PROACTIVE PREVENTION IN THE HOSPITAL

Promoting prevention in the hospital setting has challenges as well. Again, consider falls. When patients fall, a preventable problem, it costs the organization in LOS, complications, resource utilization, and malpractice suits. Patient falls are expensive. Many preventive measures have been introduced to attempt to eliminate the problem, such as established risk assessment tools. Some hospitals assign nurses and aides 24/7 to patients at high risk for falls. Yet falls remain such a universal and uncontrolled problem that CMS is now focusing on treating falls as never events. The intent of the CMS program is to make a difference and encourage organizations to improve their programs. If the process in place is not working, it needs to be reevaluated and retooled.

The success of fall prevention efforts in the hospital setting is often dependent on staff competency. Measures can be developed to reveal competency and put the organization on notice about problems proactively. Issues such as infections, decubiti, UTIs, central line infections, and falls can all be effectively prevented by the efforts and attention of clinicians and staff. Little technology is required, only good old-fashioned hands-on vigilance by a clinician working in a patient-centered environment. For example, geriatric patients are often reluctant to eat hospital food and as a result have poor nutrition, which has a negative impact on their health status. Whose responsibility is it to make sure patients eat? The typical answer, unfortunately, is no one's. And remember, all these preventable complications are resource intensive and cost the hospital a great deal of expense to manage.

To anticipate problems and to prevent them from occurring and reoccurring, a hospital must have a deliberate process. The failure mode and effects analysis (FMEA) was developed as a methodology for prevention. Unlike root cause analysis, which is a tool to analyze problems reactively, FMEA is a proactive tool, analyzing processes in order to identify potential risk points that might cause harm to patients. The goal of using FMEA is to locate gaps and weaknesses in the process of care and make improvements *before* patient safety is compromised. Because a proactive analysis identifies problems and prevents processes and systems from breaking down and causing harm to patients, proactive risk assessment of a high-risk process is required by the Joint Commission as part of an organization's performance improvement plan.

In this assessment, a multidisciplinary team employs FMEA to examine a high-risk process and develop a process flow. Once the process is analyzed, weaknesses can be identified. For example, if a health care organization has prioritized medication administration as the process to analyze, the first step is to assess whether the physician who prescribes medication has evaluated the patient appropriately. This one prong in a multipronged process has the potential for multiple errors and harm: the physician could have looked at the wrong patient's chart, ordered inappropriate medication, written the order illegibly, made an incorrect calculation about medication dosage, failed to note drug-drug interactions, or given an unclear telephone order.

Once these risks are defined, the next part of the process is to develop safeguards so that each of these identified areas of risk is safer. Taking strong proactive steps to prevent harm is a useful but time-consuming process. Often clinicians resent the time spent and do not value the analysis. With leadership support, this mind-set might change.

NATIONAL PATIENT SAFETY GOALS

The National Patient Safety Goals (NPSGs) are all about prevention. They were formulated in response to the public's demand for improved patient safety, a relatively recent phenomenon. Before the Institute of Medicine reported that hospitalizations were accompanied by tremendous risks and that close to 98,000 deaths annually were preventable, patients had more trust in their hospital experience. Now media attention is focused on how unsafe treatment is. Once the media highlighted the problem, the government got involved. Safety became a top priority and unsafe practices a national crisis.

External forces are driving prevention efforts. The NPSGs focus attention on gaps that seem prevalent in many health care organizations. If one physician does not have good hand hygiene, and there are no consequences to the patient, such as infection, it is hard to focus the organization's attention on correction. However, when the problem is targeted as part of a national safety effort, with associated measures related to improved outcomes and compliance required for accreditation, it makes an impact. Organizations are required to measure, keep track of events and outcomes, and develop preventive programs based on the goals. The NPSGs are also benefiting from the new movement for transparency of care. Both CMS and the Joint Commission require that these measures be followed.

Sets of National Patient Safety Goals have been defined by the Joint Commission and CMS for the different types of health care organizations. There are detailed goals for hospitals, long-term care facilities, behavioral health, laboratories, networks, ambulatory centers, and office-based surgical centers. The goals focus on problems; the institution is expected to develop appropriate solutions. The following list shows a large sample of the current goals for hospitals (the numbering does not reflect actual goal numbers). The list suggests specific preventable problems encountered by patients that require improvements. Organizations have no choice but to invest in finding a way to comply with these preventive goals.

1. Improve the accuracy of patient identification

    ▪ Use two identifiers

2. Improve the effectiveness of communication among caregivers

    ▪ Verify phone orders or reported test results with "read-back"

    ▪ Define abbreviations NOT to be used

- Measure the timeliness of test results
- Standardize "hand off" communication, including an opportunity to ask and answer questions

3. Improve the safety of using medication

- Develop a policy to prevent errors in look-alike/sound-alike drugs
- Label all medications and their containers
- Reduce harm associated with anticoagulant therapy

4. Reduce the risk of health care–associated infections

- Comply with the list of CDC and WHO guidelines
- Manage health-care associated infection as a sentinel event

5. Accurately and completely reconcile medications across the continuum of care

- Ensure that a process exists to reconcile the patient's current medications with those ordered in the hospital
- Provide the next caregiver or level of service with the complete list of the patient's medications
- Provide the complete list of medications to the patient at discharge

6. Reduce the risk of harm from falls

- Implement and assess the effectiveness of a falls prevention program

7. Encourage patients to be active participants in their care

- Define a process for patients to communicate their concerns about safety

8. Identify safety risks inherent in the organization's patient population

- Identify patients at risk for suicide if caring for behavioral health patients

9. Improve recognition and response to changes in the patient's condition

- Develop a method to request assistance from specialists if the patient's condition is worsening

TECHNOLOGY AND PREVENTION

The value of the electronic medical record (EMR) is now basically accepted by the medical community. However, as with the functionality of most technology, a great deal of the EMR's usefulness depends on how it is designed.

Garbage in, garbage out, as they say. One use for the EMR is as a tool to efficiently gather data to comply with CMS measures. However, if the EMR is to be used to effectively evaluate care, that is quite another issue. Most health care organizations are under pressure to develop EMRs, at enormous expense. Therefore the value of the EMR has to be carefully assessed.

Clinicians find the EMR a convenient tool. It means they spend less time writing reports and less time searching through the (often copious) medical record for information. The electronic medical record also enables a reliable and smooth transfer of information, which is especially important with so many caregivers providing services to each patient. Also, the EMR can enhance communication. For example, if the evidence-based CMS measures for pneumonia are incorporated into a patient's medical record, they serve as a reminder for what should be done at what point in the episode of illness.

Unfortunately, many of the measures taken from the electronic medical record are used simply to demonstrate compliance with regulations. But it is possible to design an EMR with different assumptions, with embedded measures of prevention. Analysts could then use the EMR database for research. For example, a national registry presently documents information about transplant patients. Our group of analysts working with this database and building on its information developed a Web-based data collection tool that addresses questions about morbidity after transplants and about outcomes. The goal of the database is to understand complications in order to proactively reduce events. The more information that is collected, the better the prevention efforts will be.

It is important to distinguish between two kinds of measures—*quantitative* and *qualitative*. Obviously, the EMR can be very useful for gathering data about quantitative measures. Was blood given or not? Were antibiotics given and stopped during the appropriate time frame or not? These kinds of questions are easily answered by the EMR, and many of the required CMS measures are in fact quantifiable.

However, although the EMR can document whether or not smoking cessation education was given, it cannot reveal whether it was effective or whether discharge instructions were comprehensible. The EMR can collect data about admission and readmission during a time frame, but it cannot capture information about the preventive effectiveness of a thorough history and physical.

The distinction between different kinds of data is an important one. Qualitative measures that are useful for performance improvement should also be incorporated into the EMR so that the information can be used for research and analysis. CMS process variables are checked for the reliability of the data collection. However, the EMR is often not designed to accommodate clinical impressions. Providing the capacity for qualitative information would add value to the database. If a patient is at risk for decubiti, data could be entered about management and which consultations were required. Was plastic surgery involved or nutrition or physical therapy?

To produce a useful and universal medical record you need, first, to incorporate basic information. Then depending on the need of the organization, information that is relevant to quality issues can be added. For example, a window devoted to central line infections could be included, with a checklist of what should be done to prevent these infections from occurring. Another window could be populated with information about patients who did develop an infection (what disease they had and what the treatment and outcome were), and those data can be compared to the checklist.

In addition to attending to design and content issues, it is important to define specifics of the data entry process. Who should be responsible for entering the data? When should data be entered? Should data be entered by the physician on the spot, or can that responsibility be assigned to another person? Organizational leaders have to think through such problems. Ideally, the EMR will be a multipurpose tool, with many people entering information. For example, if a patient in the ICU is on a feeding tube, nutrition specialists would be responsible for entering information about calories and other nutritional information, radiologists would enter information about the correct placement of the tube, once the X-ray confirms the placement; and clinicians would keep an ongoing record of infection. All this information gathered together on a database would be an invaluable tool for research and analysis for prevention and improvements in patient safety. The challenge is to define the EMR as a database that both produces statistical information about care and profiles the patient's health status.

SUMMARY

Organizations should promote prevention because

- Governmental agencies reward organizations that can document improved prevention

- Prevention reduces the financial burden of health care

- The traditional economic model of payment for services is changing

- Patient outcomes improve when patients understand preventive care

- Accreditation requires documentation of preventive efforts

- Patient outcomes and organizational efficiency are increased when data about prevention are used to analyze care

- Costs associated with managing chronic diseases are reduced

- Improving preventive care in the ambulatory setting reduces hospital expenses and promotes improved resource utilization

KEY TERMS

ambulatory care   NPSGs
chronic disease management   prevention
FMEA

THINGS TO THINK ABOUT

As the CEO of an organization in a depressed economy, how could you argue for spending money on prevention efforts?

1. What data would you use to convince the board of trustees that resources should be allocated toward prevention?

2. How would you make use of governmental attempts to impose preventive measures on organizations to strengthen your argument?

3. How would you enlist the clinical staff to promote prevention efforts?

4. How would you argue for improved prevention in the ambulatory care setting?

5. How would you measure the value of prevention?

CHAPTER

6

THE COST OF SENTINEL EVENTS

LEARNING OBJECTIVES

- Explain the resources used and expenses incurred when there is a sentinel event
- Explain how incident analysis identifies gaps in the delivery of care
- Describe how to conduct a root cause analysis
- Explain how the never event campaign is improving patient safety and lowering costs
- Explain how errors can occur in a traditional hospital culture

Errors and mistakes are inevitable in health care. Particularly in today's complex health care environment, with multiple caregivers treating increasingly elderly patients who have chronic diseases and multiple comorbidities, errors can be expected to occur. Therefore, an organization has to confront errors head-on and challenge clinicians to evaluate their care and identify and correct poor processes that lead to mistakes.

I am frequently asked to speak to medical boards about their organization's poor outcomes and serious patient safety issues. The clinicians tell me that nothing is wrong, that processes are fine, that the care delivered in the hospital is perfect, and that no one makes mistakes. When I point out that the rate of mortality for a specific disease or procedure is higher than the state and national averages, the clinicians say that is because the patients they treat are sicker. When I explain that the rankings are adjusted to account for the sickness of patients, the clinicians say that bad outcomes are the normal complication of the illness. Sometimes they claim that the root of the problem is that the coder who collects the information documents it incorrectly, and therefore the data are suspect. Generally, physicians do not want to be challenged, even when confronted with statistical evidence that there are problems in their delivery of care.

Similarly, when confronted with a serious medical error, a sentinel event (see Chapter One), caregivers are often dumbfounded. They do not know how a serious and preventable mistake could have occurred to their patient. In their acute distress they claim that something must have ripped in the otherwise perfect fabric of care. When the event is analyzed, facts usually reveal that several existing processes have been vulnerable to problems and that it was simply a matter of time until a catastrophic event occurred.

Governmental interventions are necessary because organizational and clinical leaders find it difficult to identify and correct small problems before they become big ones. In an attempt to identify and reduce sentinel events, the Joint Commission has taken various steps, such as requiring hospitals to perform failure mode and effects analyses (FMEAs) (see Chapter Five), and publishing information about sentinel events occurring anywhere in the nation to alert all health care organizations to potentially disastrous problems. The Joint Commission has also developed preventive processes that promote and support the National Patient Safety Goals (see Chapter Five), such as the "time out" in surgery. The Centers for Medicare and Medicaid Services (CMS) is also working to reduce sentinel events and has identified never events (see Chapter Four), incidents that organizations should eliminate if they are not to forfeit payment.

In New York State and some other states, serious incidents are required to be reported to the state department of health. They are expected to be analyzed for causes, which, when identified, have to be corrected. Fines can be levied against hospitals when their care does not meet acceptable standards. An infrastructure of peer review, medical board review, and governance participation must oversee the process of outcome analysis. Someone has to be held accountable for the analysis and the implementation of the corrective action. Not only does the state review the incident and the corrective action but it also makes recommendations for improvements and conducts site visits to ensure that improvements have been implemented.

CHANGING THE INCIDENT ANALYSIS FRAMEWORK

Before the recent focus on patient safety, initiated by the Institute of Medicine (IOM) report on unnecessary and preventable deaths in hospitals and the subsequent media focus on preventable injuries, serious errors were discussed behind the closed doors of the morbidity and mortality (M&M) conference. The M&M conference is not a public forum and its focus is on educating individual physicians who report individual problems rather than on identifying gaps in care or flawed processes in the delivery of care.

The IOM publications *To Err Is Human* and *Crossing the Quality Chasm* have helped to change the focus from the clinician to the process or system of care. Errors have been identified as resulting from flaws in processes. Organizations are now encouraged by the Joint Commission and governmental health care agencies to report and analyze sentinel events by performing a root cause analysis of each incident. They also recommend that corrective actions be developed once the gap in safety is identified. This process—asking why an event took place, linking process with outcome, and developing corrective actions to avoid a repetition of the poor outcome—requires input from clinicians. Analysis of sentinel events can help organizations construct barriers to avert patient harm and thus move organizations toward improvements in patient safety.

The Joint Commission offers a matrix that highlights the processes that should be examined for a root cause analysis. For example, those professionals who are involved in the review are asked to consider the environment in which the event occurred, whether patient identification was a factor, and whether the continuum of care was part of the flawed process that led to the error. Considerations such as the effectiveness of communication among staff and with family, the adequacy of technological support, the availability of information, and the accuracy of medication management are also typically part of the review.

Incident analysis has been of great benefit to the health care organization in which I work because it has encouraged collaboration between quality management staff and physicians. A communication and accountability structure has been developed and integrated into every level of the organization. In order for all involved staff to monitor processes, assess the delivery of care, and identify the root causes of poor outcomes, data were needed. Appropriate measures were developed by interdisciplinary communication and consensus. The committee structure (see Chapter Two) helped information move seamlessly from the frontline unit caregiver to the boardroom. When there are open and ongoing lines of communication, emphasis is put on corrective actions and ensuring improved practices rather than on finger pointing and blame.

To become educated about the basic tenets of quality management, board members needed time and commitment. They were unused to examining clinical care and unfamiliar with quality data. However, when sentinel events occur, board members in any health care organization want to understand how such tragic mistakes could happen on their watch. Leaders need to know the extent of the problem (how often it has occurred) and the severity of the problem (what outcomes are associated with those occurrences). Quality management data and processes stress accountability. Something went wrong with the treatment plan or the implementation of the plan. Identifying the cause of the problem, usually through the root cause analysis process, encourages the entire organization to review the delivery of care. The value to the organization resides in bringing people together to understand a problem and prevent its recurrence.

Incident analysis, led by quality management, moves the onus from the clinician to the organizational process, dramatically changing the way outcomes are analyzed. Asking why an event occurred or inquiring into what process was broken forces data collection. Every serious incident provides a platform from which to build improved processes and correct faulty ones. The underlying assumption is that there is something wrong or defective or deficient in the process of care. Blame is not assigned to particular individuals. The National Patient Safety Foundation also emphasizes the message that the system is where the error resides; it does not reside in the individual who works within the faulty system.

If the organization has proactively developed appropriate processes and staff have been educated in the use of quality management tools and techniques, many events can be avoided. Proactive analysis of care has to be methodical and deliberate. Improvements eliminate waste by changing practice. Think, for example, of the waste involved with postoperative bleeding. Usually a reoperation is required to address this bleeding. If it is not addressed immediately, severe consequences can occur. This is wasteful rework and can be avoided if the cause of the bleeding is addressed and fixed so the problem does not occur in the first place. Using a method such as the Plan-Do-Check-Act (PDCA) cycle, which requires multidisciplinary participation and involvement, results in meaningful improvements in acquiring technical skills, making communication more effective, understanding the problem, and devising solutions.

It takes a great deal of education to implement new practices. Physicians are often reluctant to change their traditional way of doing things. They may be suspicious that change will have unforeseen consequences. Reculturation and resocialization of the profession is a very slow process. Although the public now has less tolerance of poor outcomes, the peer review process still displays tolerance of errors. But preventing disastrous consequences for the patient, the physician, and the organization, especially in today's environment of patient-centered care and transparency, must be accomplished.

THE VALUE OF ROOT CAUSE ANALYSIS

As with the introduction of all improvements, unless the leadership stands firmly behind the enterprise of quality management's effort to reduce errors, it is doomed to failure. If the root cause analysis of an event is performed to comply with state mandates or to comply with a Joint Commission inquiry, it will be superficial and will not lead to real improvement. In addition to providing leadership support, the organization needs to support blame-free inquiries into the process of care. The goal in each instance is to find a weakness and improve it, not humiliate an individual. In other words, root cause analyses should be conducted with the view toward adding value to the delivery of services, not just complying with a regulation.

Root cause analyses are expensive to conduct. Many professionals are involved; the process takes time and effort. Quality management should lead the charge in convincing everyone that there is value to be gained from understanding flaws in the delivery of care and correcting them. Often clinicians are reluctant to define care as a series of organizational processes. Again, education is required. Root cause analysis can help organizations understand adverse events before they result in serious harm to a patient or become sentinel events.

Physicians sometimes claim that they have only one error in 10,000 cases. I want to convince them that one error is too many. Sometimes bad events occur without consequence to patients and the physician does not realize that he or she has dodged a bullet and that how the processes failed and where the gaps in patient safety lie still need to be evaluated. When a bad event occurs and does have an impact on patient safety, it is too late. The patient has been damaged, and the consequences to the physician and the hospital can be severe and expensive. I try to convince physicians to fix the little problems before they become unfixable big ones.

EXAMPLE: WRONG-SITE SURGERY

The Joint Commission collects data on incidents and adverse events, and aggregates these data in order to identify and then communicate common risks to patient safety to health care organizations. The Joint Commission also publishes *sentinel event alerts*, which inform hospitals about preventable events that should never occur. The intent is to promote improvements in the defined dangerous processes.

For example, one sentinel event alert (issued in 2001) targeted wrong-site surgery for improvement. Wrong-site surgeries are terrible—for the patient, the physician, and the hospital. They are preventable harm that should never happen. There is tremendous value in eliminating wrong-site surgery: the patient is not harmed, the organization avoids poor publicity and malpractice suits, and staff do not have to spend time on reports of sentinel events to governmental agencies.

Regulatory agencies have recommended safety precautions for institutions to implement to avoid wrong-site surgery, such as marking the site with permanent marker and having physicians initial the marked site. Another recommendation is that before the procedure begins, all surgical team members should orally confirm that the patient is correct, the site is correct, and the procedure is correct. Once in the operating room (OR), team members should take a time-out to verify with the documents and with the patient that the procedure is correct. Confirmation has to be documented in the medical record for compliance with the recommendation. If an error occurs, and there is no record that the time-out was performed, then the state attaches a deficiency to the hospital's performance that requires corrective action. When the Joint Commission surveys the hospital for accreditation, the surveyors trace the patient's experience and look for the documentation of the time-out in the medical record. They also conduct direct observation prior to a surgery, observing the team's performance of the time-out and the communication and the assigned responsibility for performing this task.

A time-out is a simple precaution, and yet this preventive measure is often ignored. Not complying can have serious consequences. In a recent root cause analysis of a wrong-site surgery that I was involved with, the physician had been

Root cause analysis is a structured questioning process that attempts to uncover what went wrong in the complex delivery of care that resulted in an adverse outcome. Conducting a root cause analysis also involves the organization's values. The idea is to create a taxonomy to categorize the in a hurry and did not take time for the time-out, and the nurse did not stop the surgery as called for in the policy. Both clinicians were punished and required reeducation. Ironically, a busy physician who is too pressed for time to take a moment to confirm the surgical site will spend days and days trying to redress the error; filling out forms; and explaining to agencies, administrators, and the patient's family how the mistake happened. In addition, these cases usually result in expensive, embarrassing, and time-consuming malpractice cases. The nurse who knew that the expected safety protocol was not being followed did not feel comfortable criticizing the surgeon. Her reluctance suggests that the hierarchical nature of the OR has not changed along with the effort to promote patient safety as a priority.

Another incident that I helped to investigate involved a neurosurgeon who performed a biopsy on the wrong side of a patient's brain. When we initially met to analyze what had happened, he brought a lawyer with him, in anticipation of a malpractice suit. Remarkably, however, he was unapologetic and explained that these things happen. He defined the error as a normal casualty of the procedure. When I asked him why there was no time-out documented in his notes, he said it was an annoying process that took precious time away from caring for the patient. He saw no irony in this position. I explained that the wrong-site surgery, easily avoided with a momentary time-out, was now going to use up enormous amounts of his time.

Wrong-site surgery, a devastating and expensive never event, occurs infrequently in other countries. In China, for example, patients are prepared for two days prior to their surgeries. In the United States, most patients have same-day surgery or come to the hospital the morning of their procedure. I have no data to support the notion that rushing may lead to wrong-site surgery and that extensive preparation may avoid it, but that certainly makes intuitive sense. Our practice of same-day surgery is driven entirely by economics. Hospital overnights are expensive and insurers look for ways to reduce length of stay. Of course, operating on the wrong site is expensive too. In order for a health care system to preserve patient safety and to avoid errors and sentinel events, it should integrate checklists, algorithms, clinical guidelines, data collection, and monitoring of processes into hospital care as routine.

elements involved in the incident, such as inadequate documentation, poor management, or faulty technology. The goal is to identify and address the fundamental problems, zeroing in on processes that can be corrected to avoid recurrences.

But before a root cause analysis can be conducted, several steps must be accomplished to overcome physician resistance. The first necessary step is to find a way to break the initial wall of resistance to being questioned. Physicians tend to insist that they know what they are doing, and they do not want nonclinicians to evaluate their practice. When presented with data illustrating that the process was poor and the negative outcome could have been avoided, physicians often feel as if they are being second-guessed. They say that they could not foresee the problem and that hindsight is easy. The second phase of resistance to participating in a root cause analysis is a "time is money" attitude,

EXAMPLE: MEDICATION ERROR

This example of how poor processes and procedures can result in poor outcomes is a composite based on several actual cases.

A sixty-eight-year-old man was admitted to the intensive care unit (ICU) because he had a rapid heart rate. A resident looked up the appropriate medication (a type of beta blocker) in a book and wrote the order for it. He was unfamiliar with the medication (it was then relatively new), and he wrote the order without pursuing the correct channels. The correct procedure would have been to contact the pharmacy to verify dosage and route of administration and to verify the medication with an attending physician. This incident occurred at night when the nurse manager, who might have been able to verify the medication order, was not there. Although the medication label carried a red flag warning, the resident did not notice that the medication was concentrated and thus required a dosage calculation that would dilute it. A mathematical error, poor communication, and not following established procedures led to the death of this patient. The concentrated dose was not verified by the resident or the nurse; the pharmacist did not verify the medication with the attending physician.

Of course all the staff involved were horrified. The family had to be informed that a fatal error had been made. Incident reports needed to be filed. Risk management had to be notified. Quality management was called in to review the case and do a root cause analysis. The analysis had to be performed quickly, while the facts were fresh. Experts in the field had to be consulted. Clinical leaders were expected to participate in the review of the event. Issues of competency, supervision, and communication had to be clearly defined and became the subject of intense education. Inexperienced physicians working without supervision at night, with nurses whose first language was not English, were involved in this tragic and preventable occurrence.

EXAMPLE: MATERNAL DEATH

Here is another example of how multiple processes can fail and result in a patient's death.

A young woman who had become pregnant after treatment for infertility was delivered by C-section because she was thought to be at high risk. During the delivery, bleeding was noted and was controlled. In the recovery room she was stable but had somewhat low blood pressure. Her initial blood work showed that her blood pressure was normally low so the clinical staff noted the pressure without great concern. The new mother was transferred to a floor unit in due course. Several hours later, when the nurse checked her, she was barely responsive, her blood pressure was dangerously low, she had a rapid heart rate, and she was in shock. Soon after, she died.

What happened? The clinicians did not respond to the subtle cues. There was poor monitoring; they did not recheck; they did not follow up. The nurse did not notice that the woman's vital signs were decreasing when normally she should have been recovering after the surgery. This tragic preventable death resulted in cost to the hospital to settle a malpractice lawsuit and also resulted in terrible publicity in the newspapers. In addition there was a tremendous amount of work involved in doing the root cause analysis, redefining processes, and reeducating the staff. Increased vigilance would have saved this woman's life.

suggesting that such an activity is a waste of precious time and is simply regulatory paperwork. A third phase of resistance is the claim that the patient's medical condition is so extremely complicated that analyzing the process of care requires medical school training. Once you get through these phases of resistance, however, you often see the beginning of a crack in the defensive armor.

Finally, quality management staff can explain that performing a root cause analysis is the law, like it or not, and that physician participation is required. Following collaborative meetings where processes are examined, physicians generally discover that the analysis was useful.

MONITORING BEHAVIORAL HEALTH

In a psychiatric setting, measurement systems are valued because they provide a way to translate subjective information into data that can be used to explain phenomena that would otherwise be difficult to interpret. The treatment plan for patients with behavioral health issues stresses patient interaction with a multidisciplinary team, perhaps more so than would be the case in a medical

EXAMPLE: SUICIDE PREVENTION

Out of the almost 5,000 sentinel events reported to the Joint Commission between 1995 and 2007, patient suicide was the second most prevalent, making up 12.4 percent of all sentinel events (wrong-site surgery was the most prevalent). Suicide is a particularly intractable problem for health care organizations to manage because there is no reliable diagnostic test that will eliminate or cure the problem. Also, it is extremely difficult to anticipate who will attempt to commit suicide; suicidal ideation is not a reliable predictor, nor is lack of suicidal ideation a guarantee that no suicide will occur. Nonetheless, attempting to identify potential risk factors for suicide is a worthy performance improvement effort, and developing strategies and tools for maximizing the safety of vulnerable patients a valuable enterprise.

In our health system there were several incidents of attempted suicide and successful suicide that occurred over the years, not only among the behavioral health patients but among medical patients in the acute care and outpatient settings as well. Suicide has a huge impact on a health care organization and seriously disrupts the process of care. It is devastating to the staff and the organization.

System leaders prioritized a performance improvement initiative to attempt to improve the situation. A multidisciplinary task force made up of medical and nursing staff and staff from environmental, pharmacy, quality management, risk, social services, and other areas, conducted root cause analyses of seventeen attempted and completed suicides during a three-year period; these events had occurred in the outpatient setting (including emergency departments) and in inpatient acute care and inpatient behavioral health settings.

The results of the analyses revealed multiple opportunities for improvement, especially in the area of patient assessment, communication, and knowledge. In one case, for example, a patient who had a history of alcohol abuse was not

setting. The objectives of the treatment plan can be measured. For example, data can be collected about risk reduction in suicides, elopements, and readiness for discharge. The value of using these measures over time is to identify potential problems in the process of care that can be reduced or eliminated. The goal is to reduce the number of incidents that occur.

Many kinds of problems can have an impact on behavioral health patients and can result in an incident. For example, if the environment of care is not secure and the measures fail to describe patients who are at risk for leaving before they are discharged, an elopement could occur. Medication errors or adequately reassessed for signs of alcohol withdrawal. If there had been an appropriate reassessment, medical intervention to alleviate the patient's heightened agitation might have averted a tragedy. Not only was the reassessment process found to be inadequate but communication was determined to be very poor as well. Nursing and resident staff did not communicate to the attending physician that the patient's symptoms were escalating. Finally, if the medical and nursing staff had had more knowledge about alcohol withdrawal symptoms, they might have been able to implement crisis management techniques. Root cause analyses of the other cases revealed similar assessment, communication, and knowledge deficits.

With the information from the analyses, new protocols and procedures were developed and implemented, targeting risk assessment for alcohol withdrawal. Quality management and clinical staff were able to improve the risk assessment in the ED to include questions related to alcohol and drug abuse and to develop procedures for psychological consultations and drug therapy to address withdrawal issues. A detoxification protocol was developed and incorporated into the treatment plan. ED staff were educated on the new processes and on better identification of the behaviorally vulnerable patient.

This improvement initiative met with success. Educational programs and targeted accountability were also increased. A standardized suicide risk assessment scale was introduced across the entire continuum of care. Quality management developed a database of indicators to monitor the volume of patients at risk for needing detoxification in the medical setting and to record symptoms, interventions, medical management, and use of the tools and protocols, as well as the outcomes of these interventions. The initiative heightened the awareness of the entire community about the potential risks for suicide, resulting in a more vigilant culture.

drug-food interactions may cause an adverse effect on a patient. To proactively monitor behavioral health units in the North Shore-LIJ Health System, quality management staff developed a table of measures (Figure 6.1) to track variables over time. By defining the scope of care, we hoped to avoid incidents by eliminating risk factors from the physical environment. We also focused on improving education of staff when the measures indicated that prevention education was necessary. Psychiatrists readily embraced the measures because they wanted to hold themselves to the same high level of objective performance as other clinical departments did.

FIGURE 6.1 *Behavioral health table of measures*

Example	Year 1	Year 2	Year 3
Average length of stay (ALOS)			
Suicide attempts			
Suicides			
Total number of elopements (AWOLS)			

ELIMINATING NEVER EVENTS

The CMS mandate to eliminate never events (events that should not occur because they are preventable) attaches an organizational and financial value to complications. CMS will not pay for preventable errors. This is a new way to address morbidities and clearly illuminates the link between organizational and financial processes. The goal of the CMS initiative is to control poor performance.

By making an impact on the finances of the hospital, CMS hopes to force care providers to develop better processes to control problems. Prior to the

NEVER EVENTS Currently, the list of never events developed by the National Quality Forum, in collaboration with CMS, contains several categories and several examples for each category. The following list shows the categories and a selection of examples.

- Surgical events, such as wrong-site surgery
- Product or device events, such as the use of contaminated drugs
- Patient protection events, such as discharging an infant to the wrong person
- Care management events, such as patient death associated with medication error
- Environmental events, such as patient injury associated with electric shock
- Criminal events, such as sexual assault on a patient

never event initiative, organizations simply had to show that they had a process in place for accreditation. Now, however, they have to have successful processes in place to prevent problems in care from recurring—an important difference.

Another advantage of the never event campaign is that the chief financial officer (CFO) is becoming concerned with the quality of care because reimbursement is affected by compliance with quality variables. And because CFOs now need to know about never events, they are supporting improved communication structures to deliver timely and specific information from the bedside or unit to the senior leaders. In order to track incidents of never events and develop processes to avoid them, the CFO has to become involved in clinical care. Bridging the traditional gap between administrators and clinicians is long overdue.

Today, with new trends tying payment to better quality and to never events, administrators have to understand quality. The CFO, finance department, and quality management department all share common goals. Care has to be safe and quality has to be good for reimbursements to be high. Administrative leaders need to know why infections occur and under what circumstances, and they need to invest in improved processes. The involvement of the CFO brings quality management into the C suite. Previously, the CFO did not stay informed about issues of poor quality. That was left to risk managers or monitored by malpractice insurers. The CFO might negotiate with insurers to reduce malpractice fees, but the negotiations were not necessarily based on improvements in care. Never events are directly correlated to care and now to payment. Money is a powerful incentive to change poor processes.

IMPROVING ERROR REPORTS

The communication of information about problems has not always been straightforward in health care organizations, which is why it is essential to develop an effective process for identifying and reporting errors. Reports of outcomes and reports of incidents and sentinel events are becoming a requirement of regulatory agencies. Many errors, such as medication errors that do not lead to patient harm, are corrected in real time and forgotten. Reports are not filed. But without these reports, new processes can not be developed. Sometimes errors are not reported because there is little consensus about defining a problem. In our health system we experienced conflicting reports on the incidence of decubiti. For some staff, decubiti were not considered errors in the delivery of care but rather typical and anticipated complications of elderly, immobilized patients.

CMS is overcoming such differences in standards by defining decubiti as preventable errors that should be never events. This agency is forcing health care organizations to stress preventive treatment. Prevention requires that appropriate reporting protocols be developed to ensure that data will be collected and processes monitored.

Organizations are sometimes reluctant to report errors because they might face financial consequences and a high error rate might result in poor comparative rankings. However, not reporting is not an option, and there are many fail-safes in place that reveal whether or not reports are accurate. Proper coding illuminates treatments. The law requires that patients be told the truth about adverse outcomes—for example, if a foreign body is left in a patient. There really is no choice because the documentation will reveal the impact of the event. With electronic medical records, an error will be encoded directly. If a deep vein thrombosis (a never event) or a fall (a never event) requires treatment, it will be in the medical record. There is simply no way not to report, especially with the move toward increased transparency.

In addition, every organization has a reporting history that reveals previous events and error rates. Until this recent movement to prevent errors, organizations were paid for complications; therefore those complications were documented and reported. If those same kinds of complications were to suddenly vanish from reports, it would raise serious questions about the integrity of the organization. If it is discovered that an organization did not report events as required, it can be punished.

QUALITY MANAGEMENT'S ROLE IN CONTROLLING ADVERSE EVENTS

Events require analysis. Not all adverse events are easily identified as errors. Mortality may be an adverse event (that is, the result of poor care) or it may be due to the natural progression of a disease or it may be a combination of both. If a cancer patient falls and fractures a bone, it might be because the cancer has caused the bones to become fragile. But if the same patient has been identified as being at high risk for falls and placed on a falls prevention program, and if that patient (regardless of disease) fractures a bone, the implication is that the prevention process failed. The best way to evaluate the process of care is through constant vigilance, using data to define good methods.

To minimize or avoid problems, not only should a proactive FMEA be conducted but quality variables should be consistently monitored, with control charts and other monitoring tools, so leaders can assess the delivery of care in real time. Many CEOs believe that quality management is dependent on a good financial picture, that quality results cost money. This organizational model needs to be completely reversed; good quality results in increased profits.

Regulations require an organization to have processes for appropriate screening and assessment for falls, decubiti, and pain. Monitoring decubiti rates may show that the rates are high. If so, it is important to develop a program to reduce the incidence of decubiti. If the rates are high and there is a program in place, that program has to be reevaluated or staff have to be reeducated. Health care workers have known for decades how to avoid and treat decubiti, yet they have remained a problem. If the decubiti rates are low, either the reporting is poor or the prevention program is working. Now that decubiti are considered never events, regulators will take a closer look at the accuracy of the reported data. Without an evaluation of the data, it is difficult to determine what is actually the case. Quality management monitoring provides the organization with an ongoing reality check.

Patients who are appropriately assessed can be placed in the right level of care, minimizing waste and maximizing value, whereas lack of proper screening can lead to an adverse event. A quality management process should review the effectiveness of screening on an ongoing basis and monitor the effectiveness of the assessment and prevention process. A hospital does not want patients in the ICU who are simply waiting for test results. It also does not want end-of-life patients in the ICU receiving inappropriate high-tech treatment despite their requests not to have it. Placing patients in an appropriate environment avoids waste and thus adds value.

The ED is a high-risk, high-volume, and problem-prone environment. Developing quality management processes to proactively avoid adverse events in this setting is well advised. When our system's quality management staff met with the directors of the EDs to develop measures, we all brainstormed the quality indicators that would enable the EDs to best monitor care and protect patients. Some of the measures now tracked over time in the form of a table of measures are volume, screening for falls, decubiti, pain management, and suicide risk. With such statistical measures, which are given monthly to the clinical leadership, physicians and administrators have information about how to manage their patients. Focusing on key variables that explain the utilization of the ED has implications for quality of care, efficiency, and organizational performance (see Figure 6.2).

Quality management data and analysis can help to change the CEO's attitude toward operations. Organization leaders must be convinced of the value of investing in a strong quality management infrastructure. Quality management also adds value to the organization by developing processes to predict problems and to design effective safety nets for problems. For example, if clinicians have an effective way to identify near misses, serious problems can be fixed before serious harm occurs to patients.

FIGURE 6.2 *Emergency department table of measures*

Example of Quality Indicator	Volume Statistics			
	Q1	Q2	Q3	Q4
Number of patients who were treated and released (discharge)				
Number of patients who left without being evaluated (LWOBE)				
Number of unplanned returns within 72 hours				

THE TRADITIONAL HIERARCHY LEADS TO ERRORS

For quality and safety to become an automatic part of the standard of care, there has to be a culture change. The traditional barriers that place the surgeon at the apex and the staff well below have to be broken down for effective and respectful communication to take place. A team approach has to replace the individual approach. Each member of the team has to exercise authority, respect the other team members, and learn to work together with them. The work is about the patient, not the physician. When the focus centers on the patient, each team member's contribution is appreciated and the work plan of each professional complements the work of the others. However, it is difficult to create a team, especially when the team leader may not be a physician.

Recently I heard about a situation where an OR nurse alerted a surgeon that the sponge count showed a missing sponge. Nonetheless the surgeon closed the patient. He ignored the nurse. However, after an X-ray revealed the sponge still inside the patient, he had to reopen the incision to remove it. Interestingly, the physician did not define this error as more than an incident, easily corrected, and was surprised to discover that by law it had to be reported. In such a situation the corrective action focused on the structure of the team, the roles and functions of each member, accountability in the OR, and leadership. In this example, leadership fell on the circulating nurse, who had the authority, and responsibility, to stop a surgery if necessary.

Another situation that reveals how complicated it is to change culture also came to my attention not long ago. An anesthesiologist confided to me that he knew that a surgeon had made an error, and yet he had not challenged or informed the surgeon because he needs the surgeon's business and does not want to antagonize him. The economics of medicine are that private physicians choose whomever they want to provide anesthesia to their patients. Such a situation is outside the control of the hospital administration. This informal relationship needs to be recognized and addressed as a quality issue, the resolution of which can benefit all.

Many successful businesses have found that empowering lower-level workers to ensure quality and speak out against errors prevents mistakes. Even in traditionally hierarchical societies, such as Japan, assembly line workers are encouraged to stop production to report and repair errors. Organizational leaders realize that small errors become big problems if not corrected.

Medical culture is difficult to influence because most hospitals are staffed by voluntary physicians who control where their patients are treated. For many physicians the mechanics of ensuring patient safety, such as the time-out, are viewed as annoying bureaucratic processes. Leaders cannot influence their behavior because private attending physicians can take their business elsewhere. The hospital finances depend on physicians bringing in patients. Imagine a heart surgeon with a large practice who is a high-income producer for a hospital. What will make that surgeon change? Administrators are reluctant to ask this surgeon to review the way he or she practices in order to ensure there are no errors. The challenge is how to reconcile the training physicians receive to make independent decisions about care with the respect for the team approach that they also need to have.

One way to approach changing the culture of physicians is to involve them in root cause analyses. When quality management illustrates how a skipped step in a process of care can result in terrible consequences to patients, doctors are hard-pressed to remain arrogant about their practices. I try to educate physicians through root cause analysis participation, data analysis, and discussion that is based on mutual respect and is without blame or criticism. It is slow going and the impact is made one doctor at a time. But the team approach cannot be legislated from above; everyone involved, especially the surgeon, has to become convinced of its usefulness. People have to be provided an incentive to change. There are many negative incentives: malpractice claims, government and regulatory reports about complaints, transparency rules that enable the public to view reports of errors, and so forth. But positive incentives need to be introduced into hospital culture as well. Quality data and processes help to provide such incentives. Data that can show that evidence-based medicine has superior results are effective and are in the best interest of the physician.

THE ECONOMICS OF MALPRACTICE

Media reports show that malpractice awards are rising. Consider these examples: $212 million was awarded to the family of a newborn who was brain damaged during delivery; $20 million was awarded for the failure to diagnose ovarian cancer; $4 million was awarded for a patient who was being treated for pneumonia and who died of heart failure. The list goes on and on.

Malpractice insurance is so costly that many doctors find themselves in a bind. In order to make a profit after paying these high rates, they need to see as many patients as possible. The hurrying and overscheduling that ensue can lead to mistakes and can certainly result in unsatisfied patients. Because malpractice claim rates are soaring, hospitals have to reserve an appropriate amount of money against potential claims. More cases are being reported, there is more organizational recognition of errors, and there is more public awareness of patients' vulnerability. Once a claim is made against a physician, the public can easily see that information on public Web sites. If the state finds that the standard of care was not met by a physician and that there was a successful lawsuit, the physician's reputation may be seriously damaged.

Culture change can also be encouraged by staff recognition of the devastating economics of poor care. Quality management departments should collaborate with risk management to analyze problems. When millions and millions of dollars have to be paid out for a specific error, quality management should analyze the process with the clinicians and develop improvements. If insurers can be convinced that safe processes are in place and that quality management is assessing care constantly and alerting staff to potential problem areas, the hospital is in a better bargaining position to reduce rates. Conducting FMEAs to anticipate events caused by flaws also saves the organization money. Many hospitals are moving to simulation labs and bioskills labs in order to train physicians in complex procedures and reduce errors. As new teaching tools become available, errors can be clearly defined and the competency of clinicians can improve.

SUMMARY

Sentinel events are very costly to the organization because

- Patients are harmed, media attention is negative, and malpractice claims rise
- Root cause analyses are necessary to improve processes
- Analyses of events use the time and resources of the professional staff
- Poor processes must be identified, and corrections are required
- Developing new processes and procedures is time consuming and costly
- Everyone, including leaders, requires education about poor processes and corrective actions
- Reeducation is time consuming and expensive
- Accreditation may be affected

- There are financial consequences to never events
- Efforts to change the culture of the organization may be necessary

KEY TERMS

incident analysis   sentinel events

malpractice   time-out

THINGS TO THINK ABOUT

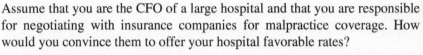

Assume that you are the CFO of a large hospital and that you are responsible for negotiating with insurance companies for malpractice coverage. How would you convince them to offer your hospital favorable rates?

1. What data would you show to convince the insurers that quality processes are in place in your organization?

2. How would you explain the sentinel events that have occurred and demonstrate to the insurers that the organization has made corrections?

CHAPTER

7

MANAGING EXPENSES IN A HIGH-RISK ENVIRONMENT

LEARNING OBJECTIVES

- Discuss the cost-effectiveness of appropriate utilization of the ICU

- Discuss the quality of care, organizational efficiency, psychological, social, and financial issues involved in treating patients at the end of life

- Discuss the medical, organizational, social, and financial issues involved in OR efficiency

- Discuss the quality of care and organizational issues involved in maintaining an effective and efficient ED

- Describe the multiple issues involved in effective throughput

Although there have been many attempts—by the government, health maintenance organizations (HMOs), individual hospitals, and chief financial officers (CFOs) of health care institutions—to reduce the extraordinary cost of health care, remarkably, these efforts have had little impact. It's time to seriously ask ourselves, Why not? Why, with all the advances in care and the efforts to improve care and reduce costs, have we been so unsuccessful? New technology and new medicines are continually introduced into health care, yet the economic and health situation remains grim. We have to ask ourselves why so little has changed.

In previous chapters, I have commented on what needs to be introduced into the culture for service to improve and for costs to be contained. First and foremost, we have to address the social organization of the hospital and reeducate physicians about how to function in a new environment. Our physicians are educated to work independently, to manage treatment on individual case bases, and not to rely on others. Research shows that many adverse outcomes occur as a result of a lack of a team approach to care and a failure of communication among caregivers. When clinicians work independently in an environment that requires coordination of care, there is poor communication and often poor utilization of resources. When treatment plans are guided by evidence-based medicine and risk-adjusted aggregated data of specific patient populations, patient care improves. Clinicians should be reeducated to value team work, rely on evidence-based medicine, and base decisions on data. With this new approach, physicians would change the way care is delivered.

Change should be introduced at every level. Administrators need to change and begin to involve themselves in clinical processes. Also, governance cannot take a back seat to the way care is delivered and focus, as has been the case, solely on financial and credentialing issues. The board of trustees needs to get involved in the daily workings of the health care organization. For example, questions about accountability should be asked from the top. Who is in charge of a psych unit, or what are the admission and discharge criteria to the intensive care unit (ICU)? Physicians should find answering questions about accountability a normal part of their practice.

IMPROVING COST IN THE ICU

The ICU may be the most expensive unit in the hospital. There is a great deal of technology, the patient-staff ratio is usually one to one, and many patients are on multiple medications that require careful and time-consuming management and administration. Patients are on ventilators, pumps, catheters; *central lines* have been inserted. Often medical procedures take place at the bedside on the unit.

The efficiency of the ICU is important to both administrators and clinicians. Administrators value efficiency because a more efficient ICU, with rapid patient turnover and a short length of stay (LOS), will result in greater revenue than an inefficiently run ICU with patients with low acuity who have a prolonged LOS. Physicians, understandably, are less concerned with efficiency than with patient safety. Many physicians admit patients to the ICU because they want patients to be carefully and constantly monitored, especially during an acute phase of illness.

ICUs are often full of patients whose doctors have ordered "rule out MI [myocardial infarction]." These patients are admitted to the ICU for observation or until a stress test (which could easily be performed in an outpatient setting) rules out a cardiac condition. For care to be more efficient, we need to better define our ICUs: what they should be used for, and what not, which patients would most benefit, which not. For example, is an ICU an appropriate place for terminally ill patients, or would a unit with less technological resources and more palliative care services be most appropriate? Without standardized criteria for admission to the ICU, physicians have free reign to place their patients in this highly intensive resource. In order for the ICU to become an efficient and safe environment, it should be controlled and managed by a team and a team leader who is empowered by other physicians to review and take action on their patients.

One of the debates that hospitals engage in is whether to have an open or a closed ICU. With a closed ICU, an intensivist supervises the unit. Criteria are established about appropriate patients and the intensivist monitors who is admitted and oversees the delivery of care. The intensivist can also help to promote efficiency of care. For example, consultations can be scheduled and managed so that all patients who require a specific service can be seen during the same time frame. Without a gatekeeper organizing the flow of services, there may be dozens of physicians calling in dozens of consultations and specialists. In addition, nurses can fulfill their responsibilities more effectively and efficiently, because they can get instruction from the one physician in charge instead of responding to the requirements of many physicians. The advantage of the closed unit is that there is oversight, someone is accountable, there are established admission and discharge criteria for patients, and there is increased efficiency.

On the other side of the debate is the financial incentive. Hospitals have to make use of and be reimbursed for the expensive services provided by ICUs. Without stringent admission criteria, physicians can admit patients at their own discretion. More patients mean more reimbursement. If community physicians are prevented from admitting their patients to the ICU, they can admit their patients to another hospital with less stringent criteria. Fewer patients mean less revenue.

MATCH THE RESOURCES TO THE PATIENT

To promote an efficient ICU, it is necessary to establish patient admission criteria. The goal is to identify appropriate patients, that is, patients whose level of illness requires the level of resources involved in ICU care. There is a popular misconception that very sick patients require an ICU. But to the contrary, very sick patients who are at the end-of-life stage of a disease may not need intense ICU services. Rather they need palliative care or other kinds of comfort care that can be administered at other levels. Research shows that terminally ill patients are often (mis)placed in ICUs; however, acuity of disease should not be the only consideration for placing a patient in the ICU. If terminally ill patients were hospitalized in less resource-intensive and more appropriate units, there would be major opportunities for cost savings with no reduction in patient safety or compromise in care.

Because appropriate assessment of patients is critical to the efficient functioning of the ICU, an objective assessment tool, such as APACHE (see Chapter 4), should be used in addition to the clinician's judgment to determine whether ICU care is appropriate to a specific patient. Physicians should be educated about the waste involved in keeping terminal patients in the ICU when resources are no longer required; they need to be comfortable recommending their patients to other units in the hospital or to hospice care.

Leadership should promote a definition of disease that combines acuity of illness with associated resource value assessment. To do this, financial and other support is needed for objective assessment tools. The government encourages objective assessment by requiring hospitals and health care organizations to develop admission and discharge criteria for the ICUs and to define the patient population in terms of which patients benefit from the expensive resources available.

Admission and discharge criteria add value to ICU services and organizational efficiency. Following established criteria commits the physician to assess the patient's situation in terms of the resources required. The criteria can be thought of as a traffic light, with a red light enforcing a kind of stop-and-think moment before proceeding. By determining the acuity level of patients, homogenous groupings can be created at different levels of care and treatment plans administered more systematically. When patient acuity is defined, hospitalists and other specialists have a better idea of the requirements of the patient population. ICU services are offered to patients based on objective assessment rather than on physician preference. In addition, defining the appropriate level of care for patients encourages improved communication among physicians, especially between hospital attendings and private physicians. Improved communication results in better care and less waste—in other words, value.

A controlled ICU, where appropriate patients are admitted for a short stay until their acute phase of illness is managed, has an economic benefit to the hospital. Recovery should take place on step-down units or on the floor unit. Focusing on the appropriate levels of care for patients creates increased accountability because the patients are watched and monitored for discharge from the unit. Without defined criteria for access to the ICU, hospitals can lose money: LOS can be overextended, the unit's resources overutilized, the unit inappropriately utilized—all with the potential result that there will be little or no reimbursement. The ICU should be defined as a step in the continuum of care rather than as a destination for patients.

END-OF-LIFE CARE

Research shows that end-of-life patients who use private hospitals undergo many more expensive tests and procedures than those patients who go to public hospitals. Having more tests does not result in better care, and it financially burdens the organization. The mortality rate is similar for the two groups.

Patients and their families need to be educated about appropriate resources, and in particular, about what kinds of resources and care are appropriate for the end-of-life stage of illness. Ethical issues about quality of life should be addressed; prolonging life at a high cost with no improved quality of life is not only wasteful but inhumane. No one wants to lose a loved one; as a culture, we are uncomfortable accepting death. Nonetheless although many people determine that if they become very ill they do not want intensive mechanical interventions (ventilators, feeding tubes, and so on), often these wishes are ignored.

Difficult bioethical questions need to be increasingly addressed as technology advances to the point at which people can be kept alive indefinitely. Families need to discuss when to stop interventions and what value is associated with intense interventions. We have no standards to ensure that patients receive appropriate levels of care. Evidence-based medicine dictates how best to treat certain diseases, but there are no rigorous rules associated with hospice care other than utilization for reimbursement.

Often the physician and the family are not in agreement about how best to treat a patient/loved one. Physicians may believe that the patient at end of life would be best served by hospice care, yet in the face of the family's demands for treatment, the physician may not be persuasive. Many families insist that the doctor do something, even if the doctor believes treatment is futile. Everyone knows a story about someone who came out of a decades-long coma. It is hard to let go. Many physicians feel that it is their job to keep a patient alive. They are trained to intervene, not to let go. These issues require open and honest communication. There are varied ways to deal with end of life. Dying with dignity should be part of the national dialogue about health care.

Patients, families, and physicians all have to communicate about realistic expectations of care delivery. The community has to be educated about what the hospital can and should not offer. Perhaps, along the same lines as the

EXAMPLE: CENTRAL LINE INFECTIONS

A common and serious problem for ICU patients is infection associated with central lines.

It was not until an external agency, the IHI, focused on improving this preventable complication did hospitals make some changes. Health care professionals should ask why improvements weren't introduced from within the hospital. Complications from central line infections have a serious impact on patient safety (research shows that 20 percent of patients with central lines die from these infections) and cost the hospital money. When hospitals institute preventive measures, the incidence of these infections drops dramatically.

The IHI reports that when five simple steps are taken, there are no infections reported. These five steps are

1. Implement proper hand hygiene

2. Use barrier protection, such as masks, gloves, draping the patient

3. Use a special soap to disinfect the patient's skin before inserting the line

4. Find the best vein

5. Check the line daily for infection

None of these precautions seems difficult or involves expensive technology. Again, we should ask ourselves why these precautions are not done as a matter of course, why the IHI must require hospitals to document that these precautions

CENTRAL LINE A central line is a tube or catheter that is introduced into the body, usually through a vein, to deliver fluids, blood products, or medication, such as chemotherapy.

Centers for Medicare and Medicaid Services (CMS) measures for the treatment of disease, the government will get involved in setting standards for end-of-life care and evaluating the role of technology for terminally ill patients.

SUSTAINING CHANGE

It's not enough to measure and to improve. It is also important to sustain improvements once they are made. To sustain improvements, measures have to be collected over time and reported to the appropriate oversight committee.

are being followed. But because such documentation is required, care is safer and results better.

One of the reasons central line infections are not prevented is that no one is held accountable and no one is responsible for holding others accountable. The managers do not set expectations for the staff to follow; the unit chiefs do not insist on proper protocols; the administrative leadership does not demand that patient safety be central to care; and the governance does not require clinicians to explain why they are allowing preventable infections to occur.

Unfortunately, chief executive officers (CEOs) still believe that quality management is an expense and that its value is for ensuring regulatory compliance rather than for monitoring and improving processes of care. However, when mortality is high and the media react, often CEOs run to quality management and say, "Fix it." They react to the emergency rather than put in place processes that would help avoid the emergency. If the CEO had established a process (or charged quality management with developing a process) for monitoring central line infections or other aspects of ICU care, pain, suffering, injury, and cost could be reduced or avoided.

This is what health care professionals talk about when they talk about changing the culture of health care. CEOs have to care about care and get involved in the details. Health care is neither magic nor art; it is a complex product that requires an effective mode of production to avoid variation and errors.

Simply put, someone has to watch the store with constant vigilance. Having the government or the Institute for Healthcare Improvement (IHI) insist on measurements helps to focus attention on a problem and helps to establish improved processes.

However, these improvements should not be patchwork. Often an improvement is the central focus of an initiative, and energy, thought, resources, and expense are applied to developing new processes. But it's quite possible that while fixing one problem, others are neglected. The full process of care has to be monitored, not only some specifics. Certainly it's a good thing that central line infections are reduced and that compliance with perfectly doable preventive measures is in the public discourse about health care practices. But it would be even better if the entire process was monitored for safety and efficiency.

For example, if the new mind-set included eliminating variation, variance analysis—the process of documenting any variation from the standard and then analyzing the data for trends—would be considered useful. Presently, most organizations that offer variance analysis as part of their quality management program meet a great deal of resistance. It is time consuming, with additional paperwork. True. However, such analysis addresses problems in processes and reduces morbidities. There is a tremendous value to documentation, worth the time for sure.

Think of the supermarket and how bar codes on products are scanned. The data that are gathered provide store managers with information about volume and profit, and also with data about what products are strong, what is selling, what is not selling, what their customers seem to buy, and so on. A wealth of information is recorded and analyzed, and information is used to make forward-looking decisions about purchasing, staffing, eliminating waste, and so on. With a defined product, such as a quart of milk, data gathering is simplified. Although health care is much more complex, data need to be gathered, which is why CMS is attempting to collect information in one place. With data, organizations can make intelligent and informed decisions about the delivery of care.

Documentation of health care services also provides crucial information. Not only about what services were administered and about volume and outcome but analyzed in the aggregate, data are also available about which processes lead to events, which patient population is vulnerable to what kind of never event, which policies are successful, which protocols are flawed—a wealth of information. Documenting care also is productive in sensitizing caregivers to potential problem areas.

EXAMPLE: REDUCING MORTALITY

One of the values of collecting data is that the clinician and organization can be informed of success and failure in relation to others. When statistical analysis revealed that a hospital had a higher mortality rate than normal for a particular procedure, the quality management department brought this information to the physician. The physician was unimpressed with the data, certain that the delivery of care was excellent. He thought that some patient death, although unfortunate, was to be anticipated. In other words, the high mortality rate was statistically acceptable to him.

Quality management professionals worked to explain the meaning of the risk-adjusted data and explained that other physicians' patients underwent the same procedure with better outcomes. We detailed the processes of care that may have had an impact on mortality and developed a database to collect information on how the patients who died deviated from the expected course of care. Through analysis of each mortality, we discovered that the continuum of care was not as fluid and efficient as the physician believed it was. To implement improvements, we created a special unit for high-risk patients and educated nurses and ancillary staff on their care. Mortality decreased.

IMPROVING OPERATING ROOM EFFICIENCY

Operating rooms (ORs), or surgical suites, are generally considered profitable to the hospital. Strategic decisions about how to manage ORs focus on efficient utilization of rooms, staff, and materials. The thinking is that if these aspects can be efficiently managed, profits can increase. Administrators stress the importance of throughput—moving surgical cases in and out in a timely way—as providing cost savings.

However, there are strong social and political factors that need to be addressed and managed to improve operating room efficiency. The operating room often reflects personal, political, and economic relationships. Some physicians receive preference in OR scheduling because they bring in the most patients or perform highly reimbursed procedures. If that surgeon is made to wait, he or she may take her patients elsewhere. Some anesthesiologists contract with surgeons who insist on working only with the members of the contracted group. If those anesthesiologists are unavailable, ORs may remain unused.

Operating room culture often doesn't permit questions. Many organizations are developing protocols, such as checklists borrowed from the airlines industry, but until the social culture changes, improvements will be slow in coming. How is it possible that wrong site surgery is still the number one sentinel event in our hospitals? Protocols are in place to identify the patient; time outs are required to ensure that the correct procedure is conducted. Nonetheless, wrong site surgery occurs. Retained foreign objects are still discovered. Unnecessary complications, such as blood clots and infection, still occur.

We should all be asking why. Why haven't surgeons changed the way they operate? Why is a systemic approach to patient safety looked upon as an annoyance? Why is a checklist that has been proved to save lives and avoid complications viewed as unnecessary paperwork? Why isn't leadership insisting that variance from the standard of care be eliminated and explained?

If a health care organization has twenty operating rooms, who is in charge of ensuring that all are functioning effectively and efficiently? What protocols are in place? Although procedures may be different and specialized, there are many commonalities: patient identification is universal, counting sponges before closing the patient is universal, and prevention protocols to eliminate wrong site surgery (such as the time out) is universal. Therefore, when physicians say their work is too individualized to be routinized, they are incorrect. Much of what is done in an OR could and should be standardized. Why are standardization and uniform processes ignored or rejected by clinicians?

Efficiency should also be monitored and standardized. If a surgeon is very slow, the patient is endangered; there is an impact on efficiency, because a slow procedure prevents turnaround time. Who reviews the OR time? Who manages shift change? Does the chair of surgery receive reports on the amount of time that operations and procedures use? Are slow surgeons identified and interviewed? Is there oversight? Structures and processes need to be developed, and

EXAMPLE: ORTHOPEDIC SURGERY

One of the most successful programs in our health care system relies on communication, documentation, and standardization. Among the complications of total hip replacement surgery is the possibility of developing blood clots, called venous thromboembolism or VTEs. One of the surgeons developed an algorithm to protect patients against this complication.

This algorithm specifies exactly what should happen, in what order, and at what time. Initially, patients are assessed for their risk of developing blood clots. If they are found to be high risk, blood-thinning medication (Coumadin) is administered before the surgery. Every detail has been clearly articulated, from preop to discharge home. The caregiving staff is expected to follow this algorithm. Each member of the team understands both the role he or she plays and their relationship to the entire episode of hospitalization. Because these expectations are so well defined, accountability is also well defined. Each member of the team understands his or her responsibility.

A nurse educator follows the patient from the presurgical office visit to the postsurgical office visit, ensuring continuity of care and effective information transfer. The presurgical evaluation involves different specialists who determine the suitability of the patient not only for the surgical procedure but also for postsurgical rehabilitation. Every patient is seen by a physiatrist who evaluates the patient's fitness for postoperative healing. Also, every specialist is involved in the postop care to ensure that complications following surgery are minimized.

This algorithm has greatly reduced the rate of VTEs even though the number of cases of hip replacement surgeries has increased. Standardizing the care and using the team approach has reduced the infection rate of these surgical patients to virtually zero.

more important, senior leadership needs to think that the development of such processes is important. If the patient is not properly prepped or assessed preoperatively, then there are holdups that require rescheduling and wasted OR time. Appropriate medical clearance should not be in any way given short shrift. Often hospitals are penny wise and pound foolish.

IMPROVING OVERSIGHT

Oversight needs to increase for patient care to become more successful. To improve oversight in our health care system, I established a high-level committee—the Joint Conference Professional Affairs Committee—to oversee quality. The committee included members of the board of trustees and clinical and administrative leadership. The medical staff was expected to report to this committee regularly on processes that would lead to improvements in patient safety and organizational efficiency. Everyone in the hospital was aware that the board was evaluating the quality of care regularly and insisting that the care be optimal. The caregiving staff realized that their efforts were noticed; administrative leaders and managers knew that their reports on efficiency and effectiveness had an audience.

Oversight can generate a culture change. When one of our hospitals wanted to introduce robotic technology into the OR, the surgeon involved was expected to come to the committee meeting and educate the board members about the value of the technology. To do so, he simulated an OR in the meeting room and explained to the board members how the process worked and how it would improve patient safety. Board members addressed questions to the surgeon and to the OR staff directly. This kind of interaction strengthens communication and creates a very high level of efficiency. The board, representing the community, holds the appropriate staff accountable. If there would be an adverse incident in that OR, the surgeon would be expected to report directly to the board members, explain the lapse in patient safety, and offer corrective actions. Enhancing accountability improves the process of care.

If board members ask *why* and *why not* often enough, care will improve. Pneumonia is pneumonia; it is what it is. However, the way pneumonia is treated, the efficiency with which it is treated, and the elimination of variation in its treatment all lead to better care and less costly services. Without high expectations from the CEO and oversight from the board, hospital processes are not controlled. If the board takes its oversight responsibility seriously and demands that processes that make the care better be introduced and sustained, care will improve.

MANAGING THROUGHPUT

We all know that emergency departments (EDs) are overcrowded. Everyone has a story about a friend of a friend who had to wait for hours before being seen and treated. Compare the EDs to traffic patterns. Imagine half a dozen highways that converge at a ramp to a bridge. Normal traffic causes slowdowns and crowding on the ramp—the sole access to the bridge. One abnormality, one car accident or breakdown in one lane of these highways can back up travel for miles and hours. The EDs address the health needs of too many people with too little space and staff. Inevitably, there are traffic problems.

Increasingly, for various social and economic reasons, community members use the ED as their first contact with the medical system. Many people are uninsured or underinsured and don't have regular physicians. Especially in immigrant communities, EDs serve as primary care doctors for community members who experience health crises. The millions of Americans who do not have health insurance use the ED for medical care because federal law requires that everyone be treated, regardless of ability to pay. No one is supposed to be turned away from an ED. Members of the community have unanticipated health emergencies, broken bones, chest pains, or appendicitis and rush to the EDs for treatment. Physicians send their patients to the EDs when they need to quickly diagnose a condition because most physician offices are not equipped with the same level of technology as hospitals are.

Many patients use the ED for routine (nonemergency) medical care as well. Reports are that more than half the visits to emergency rooms are for minor medical problems. Charges for nonurgent care have been estimated to add more than $5 billion to our national health care bill. For example, a diabetic patient may come to the ED because her blood sugar is high and yet she cannot afford medication. She will be treated, but it is a short-term solution. Without regular medication, this patient may well end up in the hospital due to complications, and her care will cost taxpayers thousands of dollars. Overcrowding in the ED reflects social, economic, and health care problems.

Inside the ED there are other issues. Patients are triaged so that those patients with the most acute illness are treated before the less acute, with the result that many people wait a long time to be seen if they are not critically ill. Trauma takes precedence over nontrauma. The critically ill who do gain quick access generally have to undergo radiological tests to confirm a diagnosis. These tests take time, staff, and require speedy and accurate communication among staff and departments. Often specialists have to be located and called in for assessment. The potential for bottlenecks is obvious.

If a patient requires surgery, then there has to be an OR available. Patients may have to wait until there is space. If an emergency takes precedence over another surgery, the ORs become backed up. If the ORs are backed up, the EDs can't move patients out of the ED to make room for new patients. The ORs are dependent on space in recovery, which is dependent on space on the floors. If a very sick patient at the end of life remains in the ICU because palliative care is full, there are traffic problems.

The space on the floors not only responds to needs within the hospital but also from the community. Physicians admit patients to the floor units for planned procedures and care. If a cardiac patient is scheduled for a specific procedure, that patient needs to be placed on a cardiac unit. Surgical patients require surgical units; medical patients, medical. The movement of patients to the floor depends on communication between the receiving unit and the sending unit. It is not simply a question of an open bed (difficult enough!) but distributing patients appropriately by condition and ensuring that the continuum of care is met. If a pneumonia patient also has an infection, such as MRSA (methicillin resistant *Staphylococcus aureus*), he or she may have to be placed in a special unit, one that would contain the spread of the infection. You see the problem. All the units are interdependent. One bottleneck anywhere means a serious traffic jam.

Health care professionals try to address this complicated issue of throughput with various new efficiency tools and techniques, such as Six Sigma, queuing theory, cost-effectiveness analysis, bed boards, computerized tracking technology, bed czars—all are attempts to address the bottlenecks. However, to my mind bottlenecks are inevitable. Hospital care is not parallel to any other industry. Although much can be systematized and routinized, much care cannot. Patients are complex; they respond variably to similar treatments. Much cannot be predicted. Patients have unique reactions. There are multiple barriers to quick and smooth throughput, and most delays are for responsible medical reasons. Many forces conspire to compete for beds, and there are a limited number of beds in specific units. It is difficult to reconcile the many parallel processes that move patients around a hospital.

Even the discharge process is complicated. Now, in order to free up beds, patients who are discharged are put in special rooms (a kind of highway rest stop) until they leave. These rooms are not patient care rooms, yet the patients require some monitoring and supervision from professional staff. In these rooms there are also delays; the room is full, or necessary social service staff is backed up. The solution for such bottlenecks is ongoing communication, supervision of the process of care, and continuous rounding on the floor to assure the movement of most patients. Sometimes delays are unavoidable because of the needs of a specific patient, and one can't automate the care or the processes. The level of individuality and the complexity of care create delays and inefficiencies in some situations. Those exceptions, variations from the norm, need to be studied to develop processes that take exceptions into account.

Administrators need to realize that the problem is not a lack of an effective queuing system or other such process issues. They need to understand the delivery of care throughout the hospital. There are well-established algorithms of care, such as pathways and other clinical guidelines by diagnosis, but there is also a tremendous amount of variation from the expected. The complexity of disease and care is poorly considered. Examples from old-fashioned assembly lines can be used to describe throughput, but in a hospital moving a patient from one station to the next depends on productive communication and implementation of standardized guidelines or clinical pathways.

Many innovations are directed at resolving these problems of overcrowding and throughput, efficiency and effectiveness of care. Specialty hospitals, targeting a specific population or limited to homogeneous procedures (for example, orthopedic surgery, hip replacement), have good results. However, these hospitals are limited; they do not admit complex outliers. There is an increase in home care patients who are monitored by telecommunications technology, which provides care at home at reduced expense. Many procedures are performed at ambulatory centers. Nurse professionals and physicians assistants are managing patients. But the population increases, and the demand cannot keep up with the supply. Also, not all patients who require services posthospitalization are qualified for such services by insurers.

Empty beds are bad for hospitals. Certainly they are bad financially, since costs are kept down if the hospital is used. Therefore the goal for most hospital administrators over the years has been to ensure maximum utilization of the facility. The downside is that now it is difficult to turn the tide and to develop a process in which a bed is available when necessary.

Administrators need to get out of their offices and onto the floor units. They need to see firsthand the kinds of problems involved in moving patients. They need to become familiar with the special units, such as the ED, OR, ICU, CCUs (critical care units), and medical and surgical floors. Oversight of throughput has to be general, across the entire hospital. Administrators need to identify barriers and obstacles; some may be remedied, others may be the result of managing sick patients. Just as variation from the expected process of an episode of hospitalization identifies special problems that need to be addressed, oversight of patient throughput from the ED to discharge may also illuminate where problems exist and where to target improvements. More important, such oversight would better enable coordination of services and improved communication across the continuum of care.

SUMMARY

Managing expenses in high risk environments involve

- Understanding the costs/benefits of having an open or closed ICU

- Establishing defined admission and discharge criteria for patient appropriateness in specialized units

- Using objective assessment tools, such as APACHE, to define appropriateness of patients for specialized services

- Understanding the quality of care, ethical and resource utilization issues involved in treating patients at the end of life

- Promoting prevention strategies to avoid unnecessary complications, such as infection

- Establishing an accountability structure for promoting safety in high-risk environments

- Developing measures to monitor on-going improvements

- Understanding the medical, social, financial, and political factors involved in efficient OR utilization

- Understanding issues involved in effective and efficient ED utilization
- Understanding issues involved in managing throughput

KEY TERMS

organizational efficiency	resource utilization
preventing infection	throughput

THINGS TO THINK ABOUT

As the CMO of a large teaching hospital, you are challenged to balance quality of care and costs. Division chiefs come to you requesting more staff and technology.

1. How would you evaluate the benefits and costs to the patient and the organization?

2. What data would you use to make your decisions?

3. How would you monitor whether increased resource expenditure was effective?

4. How would you assign accountability for maintaining safety and cost-effectiveness in your high-risk units?

CHAPTER

8

IMPROVING COMMUNICATION AND ESTABLISHING TRUST

LEARNING OBJECTIVES

- Discuss the relationship between effective communication and improved patient outcomes
- Explain the role of trust in promoting effective communication
- Describe the role of quality management principles in promoting improved communication
- Discuss the importance of accurate reporting of poor outcomes to patient safety
- Describe issues involved in assessing competency of staff

Without accurate and ongoing information, members of the hospital board of trustees can't fulfill their regulatory obligation to oversee the quality of care delivered in their organizations. Often clinicians and board members engage in informal conversation, and the clinician assures the board member that all is well. But how can a board member who befriends the medical chief of staff challenge his or her judgment when outcomes are poor? Information supplied anecdotally, on the golf course or during social gatherings, is simply not good enough. If there are patient or organizational problems in the delivery of care, there needs to be a formal mode of communication, with information grounded on data and measures.

Board members have to insist that clinicians provide them with accurate information, and they have to feel adequately schooled to evaluate the information. Accurate assessment of the delivery of care cannot be made unless the communication occurs between equals. Communication improves when (nonclinical) members of the board of trustees interact with clinicians from a foundation of mutual trust, respect, and collaboration.

With today's commitment to transparency and with an ever-tightening link between quality of care and reimbursement, board members and senior administrators require information for decision making; they are responsible to the community. When the government rankings and media reports indicate that the hospital is below the national average in important aspects of care, such as mortality and infection rates, clinicians must be asked questions and give meaningful answers (rather than reassurances).

DEVELOPING TRUST

Trust is the key issue in promoting open, complete, and accurate communication among caregivers, administrators, members of the governance board, leadership, and patients. Trust among physicians and administrative leadership and governance develops with ongoing education and frequent dialogue. Board members have realized that respectful discussion produces much better results than finger-pointing and blaming. If measurements reveal that the nosocomial (that is, hospital-acquired) pressure ulcer rate has increased, for example, board members should have sufficient education regarding quality to discuss the issue with the appropriate clinicians in a collaborative manner.

Without trust, identifying the source of the problem and defining and implementing a resolution to the problem is difficult. Board members, who have not received education about quality management processes and principles, might simply insist that the problem be solved or not define the situation as a problem. They may accuse the caregiver of not doing his or her job appropriately and recommend inappropriate consequences for not conforming to the standard of care.

Board members who have experienced meaningful dialogue with physicians and collaborated on finding solutions to problems, rather than assign blame, may ask with genuine interest why the pressure injury rate is high. Physicians, who believe that they have the respect of the governing body, may explain that certain never events, such as pressure ulcers, may be unavoidable, influenced, perhaps, by the patient's health status (for example, he or she is immobilized), previous care, or specific comorbidities. With trust, both groups, the clinicians and the governance, can focus their attention most productively on defining the causality of the problem and delineating options that might lead to meaningful improvements. In fact, it is among the board's responsibilities to oversee that the medical staff develop corrective actions to identified problems.

THE ROLE OF QUALITY MANAGEMENT IN INCREASING TRUST

Using data, statistics, and quantitative information, quality management professionals are well positioned to convince clinicians that administrators and leaders are not interested in evaluating individual performance but in focusing on processes of care for assessment and improvement. In other words, quality management professionals, through objective statistics, can convince physicians that everyone has the same agenda—improving care, the best interests of the patient and the organization. Physicians respond to data much better than they do to suggestions that they comply with measures because they are required to. Physicians comply with measures when the numbers prove that by doing so they will benefit their patients.

For example, when evidence-based medicine dictated that a specific antibiotic be administered to cardiothoracic surgery patients and stopped 72 hours postsurgery, some physicians did not agree. Their experience was that their patients had low mortality and low infection rates and that complying would upset their established and successful practices. In other words, their subjective experience overrode the evidence.

However, the quality management department was able to present evidence to change the physician's behavior. We cited the professional literature that supported the 72-hour cutoff and brought in experts to educate the professional staff. Most effectively, we presented data—aggregated and tracked over time—that proved that those patients whose physicians complied with the recommendations had better outcomes than those whose physicians didn't. Once physicians are convinced that it is in the interest of their patients to change practice, they do.

TRANSPARENCY, TRACERS, AND TRUST

In addition, the more transparent care becomes, the more trust is required from the physicians. Unless their care is always perfect—a completely unreasonable expectation—even the best physicians will make mistakes. With increasing use of electronic medical records, the physician's delivery of care will become even more transparent. Although there may be advantages to the physician in terms of record keeping and efficiency, the physician is more vulnerable to having errors documented.

EXAMPLE: REPORTS OF SURGICAL SITE INFECTIONS

Evidence exists that reports of surgical site infections (SSIs) are inaccurately documented, with reported rates much lower than actual instances. In fact, the underreporting is such a problem that the CMS and the Institute for Healthcare Improvement (IHI), among other organizations, have focused attention on the problem as a preventable safety issue. The Joint Commission, during surveys, tracks infections through a tracer methodology, and as a result issues arise as to the appropriate care delivered. The goal of these agencies is to gather information to understand the magnitude of the problem and develop corrective actions that lead to a policy change, such as administering a specific antibiotic prior to surgery and stopping the medication 72 hours post-surgery. One of the ways the government is attempting to reduce the rate of surgical wound infections is by focusing on the problem and measuring performance with benchmarked data that reflects the hospital's performance in terms of deciles. Logistics offers a partial explanation for the low rate of reports. Often, patients are not readmitted to the hospital where the initial surgery took place. Therefore, tracking readmission is extremely important to define the problem.

The primary reason for not documenting infection is related to trust. Physicians (like the rest of us) are sensitive to stigma and don't want to be thought of as delivering suboptimal care. Documentation and record keeping make the delivery of care transparent. There may be repercussions in the physician profile that is available to the public (high infection rate) or there could be an issue when the physician applies for recredentialing. If trust could develop so that physicians would not feel blamed or accused of incompetence, or worry about potential malpractice suits, there would be more documented reports. To eradicate surgical site infections, the IHI has developed preventive measures. But trust is essential for physicians to comply with the measures. They have to trust the monitoring agencies and understand that the goal is to improve care, not punish or embarrass physicians.

Any infection decreases value along several dimensions. Mortality increases, length of stay (LOS) is extended. Additional procedures may be required as a result of the infection. Patients can have reduced mobility, which can lead to other

With the drive toward increased transparency, more information becomes available, and the care provider has to be prepared to explain decisions about treatment. Unfortunately, transparency, in an attempt to increase patient

complications, such as decubiti or falls. The hospital might not get fully reimbursed for nosocomial infections; they are considered never events. With increased transparency, the more an organization reports infection, the more the public hears about poor processes of care and reacts by taking their health care business elsewhere.

You can see why there might be a Catch-22 involved in the reporting process. In order to identify problems and implement solutions, organizations need accurate reports about the rate of infection (or other problems). However, the more an organization reports problems, the more poor publicity is generated. Of course, severe infections cannot be hidden. Patients require extended care and treatment that must be documented. The issue is indeed complex, because unless a problem is identified and corrected, it will recur and possibly become even more dangerous.

These conflicts must be resolved at the level of the chief executive officer (CEO). He or she has to pressure the clinical staff to improve and report and be transparent. Senior leadership, with the help of quality management staff, needs to convince the clinical staff that giving up some autonomy by complying with evidence-based indicators of quality care will increase positive outcomes and result in greater revenue to the physician and the organization as well as value to the patient. However, again the issue is complex, because attending physicians are the key to revenue for the hospital, and they resist giving up autonomy. A hospital can develop superior processes, for example, they can have the most efficient operating rooms (ORs), but without surgeons bringing patients to the hospital, that OR becomes a financial liability. Therefore the CEO needs to increase the trust between the clinician and the administration.

Trust develops when everyone involved in patient care shares the same agenda: improving safety and eliminating unnecessary risks to patients. Patients also must participate in their care for it to be optimal. They need to listen to the risks and benefits of the procedure and evaluate the information prior to surgery. Patients need to listen carefully to information about how to prepare themselves for surgery and about postoperative expectations. Without communication between clinician and patient, the patient is left out of the process. Data show that when patients do not understand their care and their responsibilities regarding their care, outcomes are not as positive as when they do.

EXAMPLE: IMPLEMENTING A PERFORMANCE IMPROVEMENT INITIATIVE TO REDUCE SURGICAL SITE INFECTIONS

For real performance improvement to occur, the cause underlying the surgical wound infections must be understood. Problems can be due to issues related to the prophylactic antibiotic presurgery, or the timing of stopping the antibiotic postsurgery, or the type or dosage of the antibiotic. Therefore, an open investigation into surgical site infections is necessary.

Changing physician practice requires overcoming several obstacles, especially ignorance, inertia, and fear of intimidation. Ignorance can be overcome through education, and data can provoke physicians to move away from their inertia, but only the experience of trust and mutual regard can overcome the barrier of intimidation. Other barriers to change include lack of support from members of the health care team and lack of leadership and financial support to develop databases and accept new guidelines.

In order to control infections, it is necessary to have an effective surveillance system in place and protocols developed for preventing infections. When one of the hospitals in our health system participated in a project to reduce SSIs, the goal was to standardize care by implementing uniform standards. A multidisciplinary task force was formed to review and establish measurements for surveillance of SSIs. The intent was to integrate information about processes and share ideas. Their first challenge was to discuss and define the definition of an SSI. Once consensus was reached, a database was created in order to monitor volume and specific variables associated with SSIs.

Standards were developed for preoperative skin preparation with clippers, antibiotic selection and dose for each surgical procedure, duration of postoperative antibiotics, maintaining normal temperature range for surgical patients, and glucose control of patients undergoing surgery. Protocols were standardized regarding environmental cleaning, using appropriate scrub attire, using alcohol-based hand products and clippers.

Quality management personnel collected information about the variables and aggregated data before submitting the results to the infection control leaders. As part of the improvement program, the environment of care had to be assessed. Equipment and products had to be readily available at all sites. For example, patients have fewer infections if clippers rather than razors are used to prepare the skin (remove the hair) prior to surgery. But simply dictating that there should be 100 percent compliance with the use of clippers was not successful. A more successful strategy was to educate the surgery chiefs, using data showing the superiority of clippers in reducing infection, making available a high-quality clipper, and removing razors from the operating room. To promote normothermia, and to keep the patient warm preoperatively, staff needed to have readily available tools such as fluid warmers, heating blankets, and so on. Surgical sites were examined for appropriateness and to remove barriers to achieving improvement goals.

Highly specific procedures were established to improve processes. In addition to implementing improved practices, it is important to continually monitor data regarding infection to ensure that the processes are effective and sustained. Measures were developed for surgical site infection, such as the monthly rate of surgical site infections and how many patients received all the elements of the surgical site bundle (the CMS-recommended variables). Not only were data collected and reported at monthly performance improvement meetings, but the documentation was standardized across the health system. By standardizing what and where to document (for example, operative record, the ICU flow sheet, anesthesia record as appropriate), quality management ensured that data were comparable.

Data were monitored across organizations as well as over time. Our system compared the rate of antibiotic administration before surgery and discontinuation of antibiotic postsurgery across ten hospitals. When these reports were communicated at systemwide meetings, the clinicians had the opportunity to question others about their best practices. Healthy competition to achieve 100 percent compliance generated improved physician buy-in.

Any performance improvement program that involves changed practices should have an educational component as part of the initiative. The improvement project was introduced to the clinical staff, and the expectations were explicitly defined at staff meetings and in the performance improvement committees. Other venues where information was distributed were town hall meetings, perioperative coordinator meetings, ICU staff meetings, infection control meetings, medical and nurse executive meetings, and board of trustees meetings.

To enhance communication regarding surgical site surveillance, quality management sent letters to every surgeon every month to inquire about infections for both in-patient and ambulatory surgical patients. We also performed a retrospective medical record review of patients undergoing select procedures with a secondary diagnosis indicating postoperative infection. Patients were also involved. We developed a preoperative information program to educate patients about the signs and symptoms of infection.

safety, may actually stimulate defensive medicine because, to protect themselves from malpractice suits, physicians may be tempted to provide services to protect themselves that are costly to the organization and not especially beneficial to the patients. Radiological studies, for example, are used in addition to laboratory tests to support a diagnosis when one or two studies might be sufficient. At times, the use of expensive scans may not be necessary to treatment but may be ordered to bolster the objectivity of the diagnosis.

EXAMPLE: MEDICATION ERROR REDUCTION

A similar approach to that used for SSIs focused on medication errors. Much evidence suggests that medication errors are significantly underreported. Hospitalized patients are often on multiple medications, and the risk to patient safety is high. However, reports of adverse reactions are very low. Again, there is little incentive to report medication errors, especially the near misses that have no adverse impact on the patient. But without such reports, risks are not identified and improvements are not made.

When our system focused on medication error reduction, we formed a multidisciplinary medication safety task force to monitor medication errors and formulate methods to educate staff about improving safety at all levels of the medication process. Education regarding medication errors was conducted in various venues: lunch and learn conferences, grand rounds, performance improvement committees, and newsletters. In addition, medication safety alerts were posted in every unit.

At one of the tertiary care hospitals in our health care system, the Pharmacy and Therapeutics (P&T) committee created a laminated, pocket-sized card to introduce house staff in medicine, emergency department (ED), pediatrics, and surgery to best practice guidelines. The card detailed whom to call with medication-related questions, helpful reminders about good safety practices, such as avoiding use of abbreviations and double-checking calculations. Information regarding allergies, dosages, and indications for and alternatives to particular drugs helped clinicians stay current about medication safety.

Newsletters focused on specific subjects related to medication safety. For example, the value of near-miss reporting was explained and issues related to electronic physician order entry systems were described. The newsletter became a forum in which clinicians could share their ideas with the larger hospital and system community.

Not every patient with heart disease is an appropriate candidate for open heart surgery. Yet under certain circumstances physicians perform the surgery because without it the patient would surely die. However, with very sick patients, who are at end of life, they may remain seriously impaired after surgery. What value did the surgery have for the patient or for the organization? Very little. But for many physicians, action is preferable to inaction.

Transparency is also fueled by Centers for Medicare and Medicaid Services (CMS) data that reports performance in terms of outcomes according to disease. Comparative rankings are either better than or below average. Leadership has to be prepared to explain to the public what the numbers mean and how performance is being improved. It's better to develop processes to promote good care proactively than to be forced to explain poor outcomes.

Transparency is also supported by the state. For example, cardiac mortality is risk adjusted by procedure and is ranked from best to poor performer by hospital. The public has the right to know. With problems exposed and in the open, oversight will be strengthened. If mortality is high, a good administrator will work to address the problem, identify the poor practices, and provide increased safety for high-risk procedures. Without changed processes, appropriately analyzed and monitored over time, there is little guarantee that outcomes will improve and move beyond existing practices.

ESTABLISHING A COMMON LANGUAGE

What is required for identifying problems, changing practices, and sustaining improvement is a common language between physicians and nurses, based on evidence-based medicine and statistics used to determine where opportunities for improvement in care exist. The clinicians and the statistics should drive the decision-making processes for treatment. Although it may surprise some people, in my experience, objective quantifiable statistics are often open to interpretation. Often physicians and nurses do not define a number the same way or use the same criteria to highlight a particular issue in the history and physical. Misinterpretation of numbers has a direct impact on treatment. Therefore caregivers need to share a common understanding about what the numbers mean and how the numbers have an impact on patient safety.

For example, blood pressure is generally taken the same way and interpreted the same way. Because of this objectivity, unlicensed individuals (not clinicians) are allowed to take blood pressure. The intent was to reduce the workload of nurses. However, there are questions that need to be addressed. Are aides or other individuals as competent and as effective and accurate as registered nurses? Accuracy is quite important since blood pressure signals various conditions and has an impact on treatment. Are the numbers valid? A program should be developed to ensure interrater reliability and that the documentation process is uniform. Everyone involved in the blood pressure process should be educated about collecting and presenting the data.

I worked for years with a group of highly professional clinicians to develop a definition for falls that everyone could agree on. Establishing the appropriate numerator and denominator was difficult. Each clinician had a particular point of view to which they were wedded. Discovering a method to operationalize variables and describe them so that every clinician agrees on the same definition is challenging.

Typically, when a physician reviews a chart (usually written by a nurse), the physician looks for the specific numerical values that can tell him or her about the patient's condition: fever, urine output, blood pressure readings over time, vital signs. In the morass of progress notes, the most revealing information is usually in the form of a graph from which physicians can gather at a glance the information needed to make decisions regarding treatment.

Numbers speak louder than words in the medical record, and using numbers helps everyone communicate about the delivery of care through a common language. For example, if a patient has a pressure injury, and that is noted in the progress notes by the nurse, a sentence is not as effective as using a severity scale to document skin injury. The objectivity of ranking a skin injury as Stage 3 or Stage 2 communicates the information the physician needs in order to determine treatment. The same is true of scales to describe pain. Rather than note that the patient is uncomfortable or complaining of pain, an objective scale enables all caregivers to understand how to interpret that pain.

Much of what nurses write in the charts are observations about the patient that no one else is in a position to observe. If the physician is only focused on the vital sign graph, the physician does not have the time or inclination to read through copious notes about, for example, whether the patient had a headache. Both types of information, quantitative and qualitative, may be important for care. We need to establish a definition of what information is important to capture, how it should be captured, and how it should be displayed. Nurses and physicians need to work on this together.

When I have occasion to meet with nurses to discuss quality management and patient safety, I emphasize that documentation is not only a requirement but a vehicle for improved communication. Especially when problems occur, documentation may be the critical factor in understanding the delivery of care and make an impact on malpractice claims. How could an event be analyzed without information?

But the real challenge for nurses is not about how much paperwork they are compelled to do but on how important critical thinking is to treating patients. Critical thinking must be based on data, either qualitative or quantitative; otherwise decisions and judgments would be made without any objective foundation. Imagine the challenge of caring for multiple patients with multiple diagnoses and multiple sources of information without complete and accurate documentation. A good nurse, a nurse who knows how to think critically, also knows how to use statistical tools to understand patient care processes.

Nursing is a science, and like all science is grounded in data and rigorous processes. Today's nurse must be a scientist, using sophisticated data skills as well as chemistry and biology. The role of the nurse closely parallels the quality management methodology, the Plan-Do-Check-Act (PDCA) cycle. The nurse plans what to do for the patient and does what the physician and the assessment indicate. Then the nurse checks the patient's data to see whether there is improvement. Finally, the nurse reacts to the information that has been collected and communicates to other members of the care team to close the loop. None of this can be accomplished without information and careful documentation. The more nurses understand their role and the value of data, the less onerous the paperwork will be.

SUSTAINING CHANGE

Among the methods successfully developed to establish a common language is to use multidisciplinary task forces and quality committees to help implement definitions and identify variables and populations under study. The task force should focus on measurements and how they have an impact on patient safety.

Without measures, change may be made but not sustained over time. For example, with an unexpected mortality, or a higher than expected mortality rate, everyone becomes upset, and Band-Aids are placed at strategic points. But Band-Aids fall off easily, and the underlying causes of the problem remain effectively untreated. But if data about care are presented over time and across disciplines and a structure has been established for improved accountability, changed practices become more sustainable. It's the difference between reacting to data that reveal negative outcomes and proactively establishing good processes to prevent negative outcomes. To change behavior is a time-consuming process but well worth it.

To enlist physician buy-in, a proactive approach is useful. The physicians can describe their experience and together with other stakeholders construct variables to provide the building blocks of a database that can be used to monitor care. The database is then used to monitor performance over time and to set expectations for improvement.

EXAMPLE: DEVELOPING A BRAIN ANEURYSM DATABASE

In order to maintain uniformity in care and deliver the highest quality of care, the chair of the neurosurgery department wanted to develop a program that would enlist the voluntary physician into participating in an improvement effort. He encouraged a collaborative effort to design a Web-based database that would describe important issues related to patients undergoing surgery for brain aneurysms. Data were collected on readmission rates for all physicians. (Readmission might signal that the initial care was inadequate.) Data were collected on complication rates and mortality. These data were risk adjusted in order to compare the hospital's data to data of similar patients across the state.

Working together, quality management professionals and the stakeholder physicians, surgeons, and nurses defined clinical and quality metrics to track patient outcomes and follow-up care.

Figure 8.1 charts the observed versus expected mortality and complication and readmission rates (as indices) for brain aneurysm patients who were treated with microsurgical clipping, a surgical technique used to restore blood flow once the aneurysm has ruptured. Expected rates are calculated using a risk-adjusted methodology that considers patient demographics (such as age, gender) and comorbidities. Since the implementation of the database, in 2006, the observed-to-expected ratio for mortality, complications, and readmission rates decreased toward the goal of less than or equal to 1.0. This decrease reflects improved quality of care. The interactive Web-based tool helped physicians track patient outcomes and functionality, types of surgeries performed, volume statistics, and patient complications.

The database helped clinicians track patients across the continuum of care. A dedicated brain aneurysm nurse coordinator was assigned to the maintenance of the database. A Web-based prompt reminded the nurse to call patients regarding follow-up visits, angiograms, MRIs, and other procedures, ensuring that care did not stop as the patient left the hospital. The database tracked all

MONITORING CARE

The pay-for-performance initiative uses a detailed and painstaking approach to ensure that the variable to be measured is appropriate to the disease. The measures were formulated from evidence-based medicine and professional guidelines. Rather than consider compliance with these measures as an attempt by the government to enforce cookie-cutter medicine, these measures provide the common language required for everyone to communicate effectively.

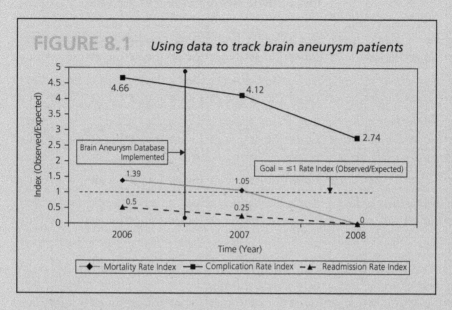

FIGURE 8.1 *Using data to track brain aneurysm patients*

aspects of the patient's stay, including patient information, medical information, primary surgical procedure, other procedures, complications, and discharge information.

To further ensure follow-up care, a brain aneurysm support group was established. Suitability for participation in the group was based on functionality through the database information. The database helped to focus attention on the continuum of care. The transparency of on-demand, real-time, Web-based reports enabled physicians easily to see a snapshot of their patients.

The success of the program educated physicians about the importance of using data to reduce variation and drive best practices. The collaboration between clinicians and quality management allowed physicians to readily compare data with other hospitals and to present data at neurovascular conferences.

Guidelines should be presented in a quantifiable manner as well as measurements. Measures reveal the distance between performance of the physician or the organization with the average expectation across the nation. This approach changes perception from disparaging cookbook medicine to embracing best practices.

Yet with all the guidelines and government intervention and initiatives for improvement that are financially based, many safety goals have not been reached. Aspirin is not administered to all patients who complain of chest pain in the ED. Even if the measure is complied with 95 percent of the time,

TABLE 8.1 Myocardial infarction table of measures

	2007 Q1	2007 Q2	2007 Q3	2007 Q4	2008 Q1	2008 Q2
Aspirin at arrival	91%	100%	100%	98%	100%	100%
	★	★★★	★★★	★★	★★★	★★★
Aspirin prescribed at discharge	78%	100%	100%	100%	100%	100%
	★	★★★	★★★	★★★	★★★	★★★
Beta-blocker at arrival	100%	96%	100%	100%	100%	97%
	★★★	★★	★★★	★★★	★★★	★★
Beta-blocker prescribed at discharge	90%	100%	100%	94%	100%	100%
	★★	★★★	★★★	★★	★★★	★★★

★★★ Hospital performed above the CMS top 10th percentile
★★ Hospital performed between the CMS 10th percentile and the 50th percentile
★ Hospital performed below the CMS 50th percentile

leaders should investigate the cause behind the remaining 5 percent. Before performance measures were required to be collected by organizations for pay-for-performance programs, the only way an organization could evaluate a medical diagnosis and treatment plan was by examining the effects or outcomes of the treatment, using variables such as LOS, mortality, and morbidity.

Table 8.1 shows data collected for four measures related to care of patients who suffered myocardial infarctions, that is, heart attacks, over time, by quarters, for one hospital. The stars encode how the hospital performed compared to the CMS benchmark. With this information, graphically displayed, leadership can quickly understand that improvements have been made in three of the four variables and can target an inquiry into why beta-blockers have not been given to patients at arrival.

Using statistics, measures, and numbers to understand care results in improved decision making and planning. Patients benefit and costs are reduced. The value of measures is being established through the regulatory agencies and the government, not by medical schools. I think it is high time to teach clinicians how to use quality methods and data to improve care. Knowledge can be coordinated with experience. The more you know, the better you perform. By quantifying care and sharing results, communication improves and a team approach can be embraced.

These issues may improve with the increase of electronic medical records. There may be fewer consultations and there may be less subjectivity because with pull-down screens for specific diseases, the more numerical information is entered the better. Quality analysts can help clinicians compare their data results to benchmarks for the nation.

Good processes have to be developed in order to identify poor processes. If good processes are introduced, then errors can be minimized. When serious problems are identified and openly discussed, the risk of repeating the problem is reduced. If even one or two serious problems are identified, don't wait for more before developing an improvement plan. With measures in place for monitoring the delivery of care and processes developed to avoid recurrence of problems, improvements can be sustained over time. Root cause analyses should be used to identify underlying causes of problems.

Working together, administrators can target process problems, clinicians can define medical issues to improve, and finance leaders may review the effectiveness of expenditures. By taking a positive and proactive role in improving care, in an atmosphere of trust and mutual regard, meaningful improvements can be made and sustained over time.

ASSESSING COMPETENCY

Some people believe that hospitals are only as good as the people who work in them. There is something to that. Yet establishing definitions of what makes a competent employee is often lacking from administrative responsibilities. Good schooling used to be a proxy for competency, but that is no longer an adequate standard. Malpractice used to be a proxy for evaluating clinical care, but today we have more objective tools. Today's hospitals and health care organizations are taking a proactive approach to defining competency in terms of requirements and through monitoring quality variables. Public report cards are helping to encourage high standards.

Important questions need to be asked—and answered. What steps can and should be taken to provide, monitor, and improve the labor force in the hospital? How can clinical competency be evaluated, and by whom? What kinds of educational programs are available to ensure that the delivery of services is congruent with new technology? What is the role and responsibility of leadership in ensuring that credentialing requirements are met? What is the financial and patient safety advantage in becoming a Center of Excellence?

Human resource (HR) departments are responsible for defining criteria for employment positions and also criteria for evaluating performance. These criteria are job specific and generic. In other words, a nurse needs to fulfill certain requirements; the maintenance manager needs to fulfill other requirements, and so on. HR details the job description and the evaluation criteria.

The Joint Commission also has requirements for competency and credentialing, requirements for the delivery of care and for those who provide the care. The commission supports a quality assurance approach, looking for clinical competency during surveys, and not simply compliance with defined qualifications.

As quality assurance methods evolved toward performance improvement and measurements of key indicators, adverse events, never events, root cause analyses, issues that affected individual competency or lack of it were included in the employee's quality assurance folder. The New York State Department of Health requires that competency-related actions related to adverse events also be noted in a physician's folder. For example, New York State measures cardiac mortality by physician; the rankings are documented in the folder. Patient complaints, from patient satisfaction interviews, may also be part of the folder. Malpractice suits often involve examination of a physician's folder.

As the quality assurance folder developed, so also did the HR administrative folder. The HR process is formal, keeping track of continuing education, absenteeism, sick leave, overtime, compensation, and so on. In keeping with today's health care environment, HR has started to measure competency, recording leadership services and educational conferences. Most HR departments have begun to request 360-degree evaluations, borrowed from industry, so that supervisors are evaluated by their staff and employees.

THE ROLE OF REGULATORY REQUIREMENTS IN ENSURING COMPETENCY

The tracer methodology documents the details of care by following individual patients as they move along the continuum. Joint Commission surveyors examine the patient's treatment plan and the physician's quality assurance folder to gauge the relationship between performance and a clinician's level of competency. For example, if a general surgeon performs a surgery and the regulatory surveyors see in the surgeon's file that he or she has not been properly certified to perform the procedure, that physician may be considered a poor performer and the organization can be cited for not overseeing physician credentialing and competency. Caregivers such as pulmonologists and respiratory therapists who are involved with ventilated patients can be evaluated by the outcomes of the patients. Were there many self-extubations or infections or prolonged LOS for this patient population? Such an approach adds value to notions of competency.

Nurses coordinate care. The initial assessment triggers consultations, such as physical therapy, respiratory therapy, nutrition, and so on, and many patients come into the hospital from other health facilities (such as long-term care facilities) and return to such facilities. Someone needs to coordinate the continuum of care. We tend to enjoy using checklists to meet criteria or develop indices for high-risk patients. But the surveyors look for the link between staff and patient outcomes when they survey using the tracer methodology. Checklists are not sufficient to provide quality care.

The push for transparency and the tracer methodology were not designed merely to ensure compliance with standards but to alert administrators to gaps in services that might have an impact on patient safety. For example, the medical staff office is expected to review and verify physician licenses. But how does a CEO know that this responsibility has been carried out appropriately? When Joint Commission surveyors review the credentialing files and discover problems, accreditation can suffer, and the public becomes aware that the organization has gaps in care and services. Without an inspection and the requirement of transparency, no one would know of the gap. Yet a busy CEO cannot oversee that all caregivers are doing their job properly.

MEDICAL STAFF CREDENTIALING

Processes have to exist, a kind of checks and balances, to ensure that there are no gaps in procedure. In order to ensure that there is appropriate oversight regarding credentialing, quality management staff developed definitions for measures to be reported to the board. In order to implement a valid credentialing process and develop an accurate profile of a physician, measures are necessary, with explicit definitions of what is being measured. Administrators need to know if everyone, including voluntary physicians and allied caregiving staff, are fully participating in hospital processes and regulations. Long before the IHI targeted infection control as an area that required careful scrutiny, our credentialing process measured how many physicians followed infection control protocols, including adequate hand hygiene practices. If a physician does not comply with the measures, the chair of the department can be alerted.

Through measurements, there is a formalized and objective process of accountability. Without measures, there would be no way to keep track of the number of applicants for various committees, and thus there would be no way to hold them accountable. Especially with credentialing, we want to define the scope of the physician. Many voluntary physicians work in multiple hospitals, and having a rigorous credentialing process aligns the physician with the expectations of the organization.

OBJECTIFYING COMPETENCY

As we get more proficient at measuring competency, we can determine whether gaps in care or in patient safety are competency related. If so, we can established appropriate education or reducation programs, or tighten supervision or discontinue the physicians' privileges. Until most recently, there has been no objective look at clinical skills. Now we have objective assessments for competency, for performance, and for definitions of the position. In other words, evaluation of competency has moved from the subjective to objective.

Regulatory requirements delineate the role of department chairs, nursing, leadership, and others. For example, the American Board of Medical Specialties Maintenance of Certification requires evidence of professional standing and a commitment to lifelong learning, cognitive expertise, and evaluation of performance in practice. The medical board is expected to review and approve corrective actions, and improvement plans recommended by performance improvement committees. The medical board is responsible for evaluating specific aspects of care, such as medication management, blood use, rehabilitation care, ethics, and service excellence, among many others.

The nurse executive is expected to ensure the continuous and timely availability of nursing services to patients and to ensure that nursing standards of patient care and practice are consistent with current research and nationally recognized professional standards. Nurse executives are also expected to collaborate with other hospital leaders in designing services and for providing care.

Department directors are responsible for defining the scope of services provided and to establish competency criteria for employees in their departments. They are also responsible for assuring that appropriate qualified staff members are available to provide services and to evaluate the competence of nonphysician members of their departments. They are expected to ensure that appropriate quality control programs are in place and to provide their staffs with orientation and education.

The chairs of departments and services now face pressure to be accountable for the performance of all clinicians, including the voluntary staff. Private attendings work independently, but the chair evaluates their performance, recommends privileges, and evaluates their folders annually. The chair assigns privileges according to hospital criteria. Medical boards usually establish credentialing committees to review physician files for credentialing. We established an algorithm for physician credentialing (see Figure 8.2) to ensure that each step in the complex credentialing process is followed. With this algorithm, physicians who apply for appointments are carefully screened to ensure that the physician is in good standing and meets all the requirements for credentialing.

For an initial appointment, the medical staff office verifies that the physician's background information is correct. After the review, the previous affiliations are verified and reviewed, as is the physician's physical and mental health. Once these steps have been accomplished, the physician submits the required documentation, such as peer reference names, certificates attesting to continuing medical education, evidence of conscious sedation training, to the medical staff office. The file is then reviewed by the director of the service and, if complete and accurate and acceptable, passed along to the credentials

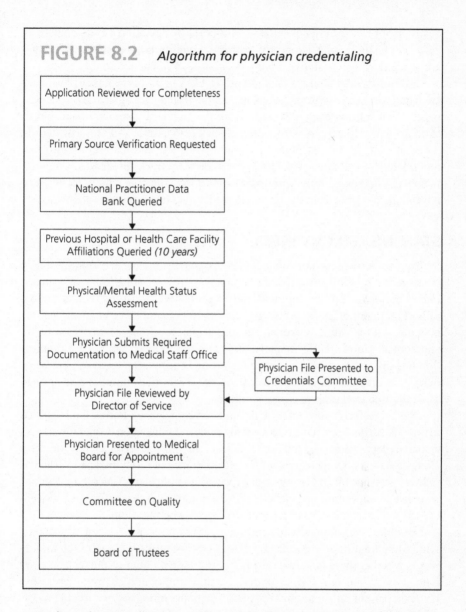

FIGURE 8.2 *Algorithm for physician credentialing*

committee, the committee on quality, and finally to the board of trustees. These steps ensure that the physician's background gets proper scrutiny and that there are checks and balances to the appointments. To be reappointed is a highly detailed process as well.

The board of trustees is also accountable for competency and is expected to annually evaluate the clinical staff. They receive information and data of defined metrics, such as demographics, turnover rates, absenteeism, staffing ratios, and individual competency. The board approves credentials of physicians desiring hospital privileges, examines reports of deviation from standard of care, and analyzes physician profiles from a quality point of view. Privileges are granted as well to define what physicians can or cannot do.

Administrators analyze data regarding LOS to assess whether physicians are using resources appropriately and benchmarking care against a physician's peers. With transparency, deviation from the standard is apparent and physicians are asked to explain. Utilization of such resources as radiological studies, scope of care, volume by physician, readmission by physician reveal information related to quality of care. Quality management tracks processes to identify which physicians comply with established protocols and which do not. If a physicians deviates from the norm, he or she may be asked to explain why.

STAFFING EFFECTIVENESS

Staffing effectiveness is a concept developed by the Joint Commission to measure the relationship between human resource variables, such as vacancy rate or employee turnaround, with nursing-sensitive measures such as patient falls. The intent of staffing effectiveness is to create a safer environment for patients. All too often, however, staffing decisions are made solely on financial considerations. Unfortunately, staff is often reduced when the organization finds itself financially in the red; staffing is seen as an expense. Yet when patients suffer consequences from lack of appropriate number and trained staff, the financial picture worsens further.

Staffing effectiveness refers to the number, competency, and skill mix needed to provide adequate care and treatment to the patient population. Generally, human resource departments screen for indicators to monitor competency of staff. Competency is often perceived to be related to patient safety indicators, such as falls or pressure ulcers, or other unexpected complications, such as infections associated with central line catheters. The assumption is that sufficient and well-trained staff would reduce or prevent unexpected complications.

But like everything else in health care, assumptions should not be accepted without being tested. The question actually being tested with all of the indicators is whether there is a relationship between the number of nurses and good outcomes. When our system undertook an examination of the relationship between patient falls and direct patient care hours of nurses, we found no correlation. The situation is more complicated, and there are important intervening factors between the falls (or other indicator) and the staff number. Good outcomes depend on many variables: an effective team approach to the patient's treatment plan, patient-focused care, good communication among caregivers, patient participation and education.

Rather than take a simple linear approach to the relationship between staffing and outcomes, we tried to educate the nurses about the value of data to understand the scope and process of care. When nurse managers have data about their patients, they can manage their staffing needs more efficiently than if the ratios are either static or changed ad hoc. Aggregated data can expose trends that are useful for middle management for planning. With appropriate assessments, nurses can locate high-risk patients and provide special treatment and processes to prevent falls, for example. Hospital care is highly differentiated, and simply adding volume to the staff may not increase competency or good outcomes.

PROMOTING COMPETENCY

If administration wants a good workforce, they need to invest in education. In return, staff will be more effective and patient outcomes will improve. A highly motivated workforce returns good results. The best and most objective way to manage a workforce is with measures that promote accountability. The more staff knows about a disease process or a procedure, the more they can meet expectations of the clinician and of the patient.

Another important issue about competency and staffing effectiveness is effective teamwork. Many caregivers of different backgrounds play an integral role in a single patient's care. These caregivers report to different individuals. What is the best way to bring everyone together? Usually evaluations are not based on team performance but on individual performance. Everyone is evaluated by his or her own director. But effective communication cannot be measured in isolation.

With the introduction of evidence-based medicine into patient care, nurses have criteria available about what steps to take, in what order, to best provide care. If a hospital or health care organization wants to be recognized as excellent, it needs to have published rankings of good results. For example, at a stroke center, there has to be documentation that nurses have the appropriate training to perform a good assessment and know and follow the guidelines of the American Heart Association.

SUMMARY

Patient outcomes improve when there is effective communication. Effective communication involves

- Leadership commitment to obtaining accurate information from all levels of staff

- Educating board members and leadership about quality management principles

- Understanding the relationship between transparency and trust

- Understanding the relationship between reporting poor outcomes and improved patient care

- Accurate reporting of poor outcomes, medical errors, and near misses

- Understanding the reasons for inaccurate reports of poor outcomes

- Involving multidisciplinary task forces and quality data in improvement efforts

- Ensuring that nurses and physicians learn to report accurate information to each other in the most effective and useful ways

- Ensuring competency of staff through objective measures

- Coordinating staffing decisions with patient safety data

KEY TERMS

competency   staffing effectiveness
credentialing   trust
performance improvement

THINGS TO THINK ABOUT

As the CFO of a large health care organization, the nurse executives come to you to request more staff to provide patient care.

1. How would you evaluate their request?

2. How would you assess staffing needs?

3. What processes would you use to link staff to patient outcomes?

4. What nursing care measures would you use to determine staffing needs?

5. How would you respond to media reports that your hospital is working with a severe nursing shortage that is having an impact on patient care?

9

PROMOTING A SAFE ENVIRONMENT OF CARE

LEARNING OBJECTIVES

- Describe the scope of the environment of care

- Discuss the importance of using multidisciplinary teams to communicate issues of environmental safety

- Explain how the environment might have a negative and positive influence on clinical care

- Discuss reasons to involve the CFO, clinicians, quality management, engineering, and safety personnel in designing patient care areas

- Describe the value of using measures to monitor the safety of the environment

Most discussions of patient safety focus on the clinical issues involved in the delivery of care. However, patient safety can be seriously compromised if the environment in which the care takes place is not properly maintained. Health care services are housed in environments that are prone to problems. The lights go out, the air filters get clogged, the elevators malfunction, the smoke alarms go off, the floors are wet and patients fall—the possibilities for emergencies are too numerous to count.

Weather has an impact on care, as do natural disasters such as fire, floods, hurricanes, and so on. Employees can be injured because of accidents in the environment, such as hazardous waste material not properly disposed of or inadvertent sticks with a sharp instrument that has been used to treat a patient. The scope of the environment of care is varied, complex, and large. Managing the environment of care includes managing hazardous materials, facilities maintenance and construction, MRIs, laser and radiation safety, utilities, equipment, ergonomics, waste management, safety education, disaster preparedness, security, employee health, product recalls and alerts, fire safety—and more. Clearly, many specialists, professionals, and staff are involved in maintaining the hospital environment.

As health care environments change, vigilant efforts are needed to ensure patient safety and the safety of the health care worker. The current health care environment poses tremendous risks to patients, and a proactive, multidisciplinary approach is needed to address the safety needs of patients and staff. Diagnostic and therapeutic uses of lasers, radiation, radioactivity, and clinical monitoring devices present hazards. It is important that patient safety keep up with technological advances. Therefore, monitoring patient safety in new environments is important to mitigate risk. Too often, danger is only realized after an event or incident occurs, not proactively.

An example of how environmental issues affect patient and employee safety involves radiation. A nuclear medicine patient was injected for a bone scan and some radioactive material spilled during the procedure. The contamination was only discovered two hours later when the patient was sent for an imaging test. The patient was decontaminated and the scan was performed. But additional contamination was identified in the radiology department and the injection room had to be closed for decontamination for a day. One technologist was sent home due to contamination of her street clothes, and all technologists were retrained about safety practices.

COMMUNICATION ACROSS DISCIPLINES

Not only do those who manage different aspects of the environment need to communicate with each other, but they also need to communicate with the clinical staff and with hospital administrators.

Physicians focus on the medical problems of their patients and how to best resolve them, and it is the responsibility of the hospital staff to support their efforts. Physicians do not feel responsible for maintaining a safe environment; someone else is charged with doing so. Yet harm can come to patients if physicians remain outside the team that maintains the environment of care. Physicians need to learn about the environment from the support staff and from nonclinicians; yet physicians who are typically in authority positions are not easily taught by staff. Also, physicians may be impatient with education about the environment of care, or how to properly dispose of sharps or what to do in case of a power failure. In my experience, quality management personnel can mediate between the physician and staff by providing education and setting the stage for interaction by forming task forces, especially around incidents that harmed patients because of problems in the environment.

Just as the physicians need to learn the role of the environment in maintaining patient safety, those individuals who are responsible for the environment need to understand the relationship of the environment to good clinical outcomes. The environment should be assessed by a multidisciplinary group, because each group takes its perspective to the table. For example, when an operating room (OR) was being designed, physicians met with the engineers to figure out where and how many outlets were required to accommodate the needed equipment without interfering with the team's movements. The design also needed to respond to efforts to minimize the opportunity for infection to develop. Quality management and infection control professionals collaborated with the architect, physicians, and engineers. Together, we ensured that there would be easy access to the equipment, that the airflow could be monitored, and that sterilization processes would not be compromised.

The chief financial officer (CFO) also needs to be involved with the professionals who are designing patient care units because he or she needs to understand how to budget resources for infection control, adequate airflow, backup generators, and so on. Safety officers should be involved in the planning stages of any construction or renovation.

Communication should be encouraged among people who previously had little communication and were divided by distinct and seemingly unrelated areas of responsibilities. Through collaboration, they begin to share a common language. Administrators also need to become involved in managing the environment and become educated about its impact on patient safety in order to make intelligent decisions about how to build structures, or house equipment properly, or invest in expansion. There is no value to a hospital to receive bad publicity when patients are discharged with hospital-acquired infections or have suffered from an unclean or unsafe environment.

Think of the risks to patient safety that can occur due to lack of communication. For example, when I was examining architectural plans for a new intensive care unit (ICU) space, I noticed that although the blueprints were almost completed, the architect had neglected to allocate any space for sinks. When I asked the architect how the clinicians were supposed to wash their hands, he realized his mistake. Those kinds of mistakes, if not corrected, can cost the organization money in rework. Unfortunately, the people who manage the building and facilities do not generally have the opportunity to interact with the clinical staff about decision making. Therefore a structure for effective communication needs to be developed and deployed.

Some aspects of the environment that the team should think about regarding reducing infection might include, Do patients who are housed in single rooms have less chance of acquiring infection (especially airborne) than patients who are housed together, either in double or more rooms? Does placing new electronic data entry machines in patient rooms pose any risk to patient safety, or would there be less risk of infection if computers were kept in the nursing stations? What kinds of carpet repel dust and organisms that can cause infections or irritations? Are the air filters adequate to clean the air? In designing the environment, is it of concern that the patient be visible to the nursing station? Are obstacles minimized to minimize patient falls?

To reduce or prevent infections, preventive measures and proactive processes should be developed. Clinicians should have easy access to sinks, but sinks are not the only safety issue. The containers of washing solution and disinfectant should be monitored so that they are not left empty. In terms of maintaining a safe environment, a quality control approach helps to ensure that everything works efficiently. Even alcohol-based sanitizers can be a safety risk because they are flammable. The national fire protection association recommends safety requirements for alcohol hand sanitizers located in corridors. They suggest that the corridor be at least 6 feet wide, and that dispensers be placed 4 feet apart. Other safety precautions are that dispensers should not be installed over electrical outlets; and if installed on carpeted surfaces, they should only be where there are sprinkler smoke devices.

WORKING TOGETHER TO IDENTIFY AND SOLVE PROBLEMS

Using tools such as failure mode and effects analysis (FMEA; see Chapter Five) to anticipate problems and put in place appropriate safety measures can focus attention on the importance of the environment. At our health care system, to ensure that the environment is safe, rounds are conducted on the hospital units to assess cleanliness, safety, adequacy of sterile procedures in order to monitor the environment and equipment on an interdisciplinary and ongoing basis.

Proactively and preventively, rounds should be conducted on every unit with staff from the environment of care, engineering, safety, and clinical staff. These multidisciplinary rounds help to ensure a safe environment and to eliminate cumbersome processes. If a light bulb goes out, and a nurse has to fill out a requisition form and process it before a replacement is made, that is inefficient. Through rounds, where maintenance staff and clinicians can identify and correct problems immediately, a better, more efficient process can be established. Appropriate documentation and paperwork can follow. Vigilance regarding a safe environment must be ongoing and constant; once a month is not enough to maintain safety. Rounds using a proactive risk assessment tool quickly identify the level of risk and also what needs to be accomplished to reduce the risk.

IMPROVING PROCESSES

In maintaining the safe environment in a large, complex, fifteen-hospital health care system, with institutions of different sizes and different cultures, my goal was to establish a method that would create consistency across all the hospitals and standardize measurements for monitoring a safe environment. To that end, I established a multidisciplinary task force that examined deficits in the environment, using the regulatory agencies' accreditation standards. The task force included the director of the environment of care and engineering staff members. Clearly, if machines break down or there is a power failure, there is a huge impact on patient outcomes. Especially in high-risk environments, such as the ICU, equipment needs to be maintained and there should be an established safety net, with a defined accountability structure.

Measures to monitor the safety of the environment were developed by the multidisciplinary team. Working together and communicating in a committee structure encourages a fuller appreciation of potential safety risks and enhances communication among different providers. Monitoring the environment on an ongoing basis is critical because good equipment is not necessarily sufficient to ensure patient safety. A procedure for using the equipment, and education, must also be available. For example, patient beds can be outfitted with adequate alarms to alert clinicians if a patient falls, but often the alarms are so constant and annoying that the clinicians turn them off. The equipment is fine, but the process is not. Engineers and clinicians together need to meet to develop a solution to the problem.

Another simple safety precaution requires written permits for ceiling work, such as that performed by plumbers, electricians, telephone and computer technicians. These activities have the potential to disrupt the integrity of fire and smoke walls and can cause concern for hospitals when work is not monitored effectively. The permits increase oversight by facility directors.

Infant abduction alarms were designed to protect infants from abduction. But often the alarms don't function properly. With too many false alarms, staff can stop paying attention, assuming an alarm to be yet another false one. This is extremely dangerous. When it came to our attention that the number of false alarms was causing clinicians to turn a deaf ear, we took precautions to assess the proper working of the alarms.

MONITORING SAFETY

All the facilities in the system report quarterly on standards for safety, security, hazardous materials and waste, emergency preparedness, life safety, medical equipment, and utility systems. Indicators for safety and the environment of care are reported on a systemwide table of measures (see Figure 9.1), so that hospitals can benchmark against each other and improve. By tracking and reporting these measures, leadership has information about the environment and can prioritize safety initiatives. The intent of the reports is to track and trend potential and actual problems and to develop corrections.

FIGURE 9.1 *Safety and environment of care table of measures*

Example	Q1-2008	Q2-2008	Q3-2008	Q4-2008
Fire Prevention/Life Safety Drills				
Hazardous Materials and Waste Management				
Environment of Care Knowledge and Awareness				
Security Management				
Utility Systems Management				
Radiation Safety				

The primary categories reviewed include such items as fire safety drills and incidents, hazardous materials incidents, environment of care knowledge and awareness, safety management, sharps injuries, security management, incidents, equipment management, utility systems management, radiation safety, occupational safety, lost time.

EXAMPLE: SHARPS SAFETY

Definitions of measurements are standardized so that all facilities report the same issue the same way. For example, sharps injuries rate is defined as the total number of percutaneous injuries X 100 divided by daily occupied beds. In their reports, facilities specify the source of the injury. Yearly reports are generated about the type of activity that was related to the sharps injury. For example, Figure 9.2 shows that, for 2008, injuries occurred as a result of surgical procedures, blood drawing, cleaning up, and so on. A task force addresses incidents associated with inappropriate disposal or placement of sharps. The task force includes representatives from safety, environmental services, employee health, infection control, laundry, and nursing.

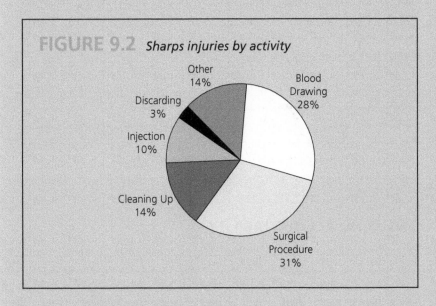

FIGURE 9.2 *Sharps injuries by activity*

New employees and residents frequently do not dispose of sharps appropriately. During orientation, the data regarding the activity that injuries occurred can be provided to alert new members of the staff about protecting themselves.

EXAMPLE: POWER OUTAGE

Power outages pose particular problems because they occur for various reasons and are generally out of the control of the hospital. Local power companies are responsible. These next examples are typical of the kinds of problems encountered and of the solutions proposed.

There was a massive power outage in the region of one of our tertiary hospitals. In order to repair the damage, the electrical company, Con Edison, had to shut down the electrical feeds to the hospital. Doing so caused all the power to fail. The emergency generators kicked in and supplied power, and there were no adverse patient consequences.

However, there was a failure of communication in that the hospital administration had great difficulty reaching Con Ed personnel because the telephone system had failed as a result of the power failure. After this incident, improvements were implemented. Now the hospital administrators have the names, telephone, cell, and pager numbers for the Con Ed officials. A backup telephone system is being evaluated.

Another power failure knocked out power to several hospitals in the health system. In this case, the emergency generators failed to operate and there was no power for nearly an hour. What could have been a catastrophe was averted by the quick response of hundreds of hospital personnel and also of the city Office of Emergency Management.

After this incident, the administrative and quality staff convened a task force comprised of representatives from the health system's disaster committee and other individuals involved in the power failure. They reviewed the technical aspects of the event and performed a root cause analysis. Recommendations from the analysis included creating multiple redundancy for the fuel feeders to the generators, hiring an independent engineering firm to assess power distribution and recommend improvements, improving communication with Con Edison,

ENSURING ACCOUNTABILITY

Ongoing maintenance is also an issue. Unless someone is accountable, problems can arise. Regular maintenance schedules were established to anticipate problems and make corrections. Each hospital worked with the local power and electric companies to assure there would be quick response and constant power. These meetings helped everyone involved to understand problems. Staff from throughout the system met and compared actions.

The system facility directors have developed a tool to measure individual competency in utilities management. This standardized form includes a site plan review and a list of questions regarding key services, such as electrical, performing disaster drills, installing battery-powered lights in high-risk areas, reviewing the need for battery back up for life supports and other essential medical equipment. All these recommendations were implemented within 2 months.

Generator maintenance was recognized as an important patient safety issue and new policies were instituted. The hospital electrician and a staff member are expected to test the generators weekly during each of the three shifts. Each member of the staff is expected to complete a self-study course about emergency power systems. Staff was given an in-service program on generator maintenance and became accountable for checking certain gauges. Nurses received education about the power supply, generators, and devices that are connected to emergency power. A new and improved manual for the environment of care incorporated lessons learned in lay terms. Generators are now tested for 2 hours at full load to allow an evaluation of egress lighting, fire alarms, and life support load. Batteries are replaced regularly according to a schedule. The Emergency Generators Performance Improvement Initiative resulted in a 10-point plan of action designed to minimize the likelihood of generator failure or power-related incidents. All the hospitals in the health system were required to comply.

Another power failure occurred when the entire east coast had an enormous blackout (August 14, 2003). Fifty-four of 55 generators had no problems. However, the failed generator had not been checked under blackout conditions, as it should have been according to hospital policy. Each of the health system facilities submitted a critique of the event, identifying areas for improvement. Although patient safety was maintained, the massive power outage drew attention to some trouble spots, such as power to CT scans and sterilization areas. At one of the nursing homes, administrative offices had no power. At another hospital, computer services went down. In some critical areas of several hospitals, air conditioning was found not to be on emergency services. Staff was not used effectively. Each facility was expected to make improvements.

water, oxygen, fire, sewer, medical gas, and elevators. Department directors are expected to review the questions with each employee and, if needed, to provide education.

Measures were developed by the engineers who best understood the optimal outcomes. In this way, the engineers, generally removed from the clinical staff, became integrated into the caregiving team. They understood their role in preserving patient safety. Generally, these individuals spend their time in the belly of the organization. When brought to the surface, so to speak, they interacted with their peers, developed healthy competition about best practices, and participated with clinicians in decision making for ensuring a safe environment for patients. The clinical implications of machinery in the therapeutic environment became apparent to them.

MAINTAINING A SAFE ENVIRONMENT

It is insufficient simply to put showerheads in hospitals in case of fire. They have to be tested; if they are broken, someone has to know about it and fix it. Accountability is key to maintaining a safe environment.

The environment of an organization with very limited resources was so poor that clinicians expected to see rodents on the floor. That's simply the way it was and always had been. There were fruit flies in the patients' rooms. Exterminators had been called in to eliminate the problem, but their efforts were unsuccessful. A root cause analysis to determine where the flies were coming from or how the rodents had access had not been performed. It wasn't rocket science. I noticed that there were no screens on the windows. And patients who wanted air opened their windows. The flies flew in.

Investigation showed that the rodents were gaining access to the floors because a breakdown in an old piping system had remained unnoticed. Once the issue was identified, contractors were called in to fix the pipes and seal off the holes. Again, the clinicians were complacent about the problems, assuming they were unfixable. They should have been outraged to work in such conditions. They didn't know who was accountable for such problems. I introduced the environment of care staff to the medical board and initiated a dialogue. By integrating the person responsible for the environment into the clinical aspects of the organization, that person felt an increased pride and sense of responsibility.

ESTABLISHING OVERSIGHT

Because accountability and communication are so crucial to maintaining a safe environment, in our health care system I developed a board-level committee devoted to safety and the environment of care. This committee was part of the quality communication structure and assumed oversight for the environment. The committee included trustees, the senior vice president for quality management, the chief medical officer, safety officers, directors of engineering, safety, and biomedical engineering, medical directors, administrators, nursing executives, and performance improvement coordinators from across the system facilities.

Through leadership, the system created a proactive approach to enable a rapid and comprehensive response to any incident, as well as ongoing surveillance, education, and training of patients, families, and staff. Using the structure of the Performance Improvement Coordinating Group (PICG), the environment of care committee reported incidents and corrective actions to the multidisciplinary group to alert members to problems and their solutions.

COMMUNICATING ABOUT SAFETY

Multidisciplinary teams developed standards for the environment and measures were defined. Reports of measures were presented regularly to the board, who became educated about the full scope of safety and environmental issues. They also became educated about the financial consequences of an unsafe environment. Fires, floods, generator failures, power outages are very costly to the organization. Infection increases (length of stay) LOS. We established proactive processes to anticipate problems before they occurred.

Prevention reduces problems and costs. If safety protocols are not observed in the MRI suite, or patients have skin problems because appropriate mattresses are not available, it costs. But in order to prevent problems, someone has to be paying attention, and more than that, there has to be a process to maintain accountability for safety. Ongoing maintenance saves the organization money. Patients who are cared for in a safe and respectful environment do better and recover more quickly than others.

By forming a board-level committee, there was a specific focus on a safe environment, and a formal process for communication about issues related to the environment. There was improved education and processes developed to teach staff to oversee a safe environment. Questionnaires were developed to test safety awareness and involved different areas, from sharp injuries to radiation to disaster preparedness. And since staff were accountable to the board for the safety of the environment and there were defined expectations to be met, there was an increased awareness and respect for maintaining a safe environment.

Reports to the board cover a variety of topics. For example, in the wake of the 2001 attacks on the World Trade Center in New York, the network emergency management group formed a committee to oversee safety. Called the Critical Infrastructure Protection Committee, its mission was to develop methods to deter or prevent critical infrastructure from being damaged by natural causes, such as weather-related emergencies, or by hazardous materials, accidents, or intentional damage. The committee routinely analyzes the vulnerability of critical infrastructure and makes recommendations for improvements.

To best coordinate care among the multiple facilities of the health system in the event of a disaster, a command center was set up to facilitate communication and to deploy resources to maintain safety across the system. Having a process in place helps to avoid chaos. Avoiding chaos in case of a problem helps to maintain patient safety and reduce costs for the organization. If an alarm goes off as expected or an evacuation plan is rehearsed, there is less chance of a problem occurring during a real emergency. When the environment is compromised, for example, if there is a break in the sterility in the OR or the ICU, it is very costly.

ASSESSING AND IMPROVING THE ENVIRONMENT

Using various methods to improve and monitor safety proactively identifies risk and results in process redesign, new policies, procedures, guidelines, and quality control programs. In addition, staff awareness of the potential risks associated with introducing new or updated technology is heightened through educational programs, newsletters, and committee reports.

For example, one of the Joint Commission's National Patient Safety Goals in 2002 was to evaluate the effectiveness of clinical alarms. Clinical alarms warn caregivers of immediate potential danger to patients. For alarms to be effective, they must be accurate and easily interpreted and appropriately acted on by clinicians. Today, clinical alarm effectiveness has been incorporated into the Joint Commission's standards. Our system determined to take a proactive approach to assessing the effectiveness of clinical alarms.

A task force comprised of medical staff, nursing, biomedical engineering, safety, and quality management reviewed the existing systems in one of the tertiary care hospitals and interviewed staff. A clinical alarm effectiveness assessment tool was developed to identify potential system failures (see Figure 9.3).

The assessment records whether the alarm was audible and at what distance. The assessment also asks for information about competing noise and has an opportunity for users to suggest improvements. Guidelines in applying clinical alarm safety were developed so that clinical directors could implement them in their specific clinical environments. Staff knowledge and awareness of clinical alarm effectiveness was incorporated into an existing environment of care performance measurement system.

Another technological advance that required evaluation was the introduction of the MRI into the ORs to aid in the surgical management of patients with brain tumors. A multidisciplinary team convened to perform an FMEA

FIGURE 9.3 *Clinical alarm effectiveness assessment tool*

DATE: _____

NAME: _____

DEPT/UNIT: _____

sample question

Describe how far away you stepped from the equipment/item, and in each case, whether you could hear the alarm:

Distance _____ Could you hear the alarm? _____

Distance _____ Could you hear the alarm? _____

Distance _____ Could you hear the alarm? _____

to prevent any adverse incidents. Hazards in the environment and potential safety risks were identified. To ensure that MRIs were safe, several screening tools were developed. Patients are asked questions that might have an impact on their safety; any issues that might compromise safety are brought to the attention of the physician. By standardizing these questions, staff is focused on potential risks.

To protect potentially suicidal patients from risk, an assessment tool was developed to ensure a safe environment. Standards for all health care facilities include securing medications and hazardous chemicals and ensuring that windows cannot be opened more than 6 inches. In the behavioral health setting, there are more stringent standards. Lamps must be shatterproof and ceilings of monolithic construction. Again, through assessing and monitoring the environment for safety hazards, staff is focused on maintaining a safe environment.

Sometimes unanticipated incidents result in the development of new processes. At one of our hospitals a hazardous materials battery exploded. There were no injuries, and the Duracell Company suggested that discarded batteries be placed in special packaging to prevent metal portions from coming into contact with other metal. A group of stakeholders developed a protocol to dispose of used batteries safely.

To ensure safety in the environment, hospitals interact with regional organizations, such as power and electrical, state emergency operations, fire departments, and so on. Communication among these organizations should be promoted on an ongoing basis. Exercises led by the state health department tests communication and coordination of activities among state and local health departments, offices of emergency management, and hospitals. The movement of strategic pharmaceuticals and medical supplies from federal to state locations, to regional points of distribution, and finally to the hospital are tested during these drills.

SUMMARY

Patient safety is affected by the environment of care. Promoting a safe environment involves

- Defining the scope of issues involved in environmental safety
- Enlisting multidisciplinary teams to oversee environmental safety issues
- Educating engineers and safety officers about the impact of the environment on clinical care
- Educating physicians and nurses about effective maintenance of the environment
- Defining accountability for a safe environment

- Involving the CFO and quality management in decisions about how to design patient care areas

- Doing multidisciplinary rounds of patient units to assess the environment of care

- Developing a proactive approach to assessing risks in the environment

- Defining measurements for ongoing monitoring of the safety of the environment

- Standardizing safe processes

- Developing ties to appropriate community organizations to maintain safety in an emergency

- Ensuring that reports regarding safety variables are communicated throughout the organization and to the board of trustees

 ## KEY TERMS

accountability   environment of care
clinical alarms   multidisciplinary teams

 ## THINGS TO THINK ABOUT

You are a senior administrator in a large health care system and receive reports from risk management that the number of needlestick injuries has not decreased and that employees are taking days off because of these injuries.

1. How can you alleviate this problem?

2. Which members of the staff would be involved in assessing the situation?

3. How would you initiate improvements?

4. What measurements would you use to define the problem and assess improvements?

5. What would the role of leadership be in the improvement initiative?

6. How would you gauge the success of the initiative?

CHAPTER

10

CONCLUSION

Throughout this book I have tried to make the case for associating quality care, good outcomes, and financial success. The more understanding health care leaders have about the process of care, the more accountability we impose on physicians, and the more we focus on critically defining the results of interventions, the more likely it will be that waste will be reduced and organizations will see financial gains. The word *waste* requires definition. For some health care professionals, waste is perceived in terms of inappropriateness of care (excess tests, duplication of certain exams). For others, waste might be related to utilization of products, such as a supply of special beds to be used as the need arises. Reoperation can be seen as waste if a second procedure is necessitated by a failure of the first surgery. Organizations can create efficiencies and add value to the delivery of care by carefully defining waste.

From the process point of view, value comes when risk points are identified and safety and/or clinical measures are defined and implemented. Understanding risk requires that processes be analyzed for defects, proactively through failure mode and effects analysis (FMEA) or retroactively through root cause analyses, and once identified, corrected and improved. Correcting faulty or unsafe processes involves multidisciplinary teams of stakeholders who meet and discuss improvements. Quality management helps the team with defining measures for improvements, collecting data about the improvements, analyzing the data, and reporting it out over time to assess whether the improvements have been effective and sustained. A deliberate methodology for improvement, such as the Plan-Do-Check-Act (PDCA), formalizes and standardizes this complex process of performance improvement.

From an economic and social point of view, value focuses attention on the patient as an informed consumer of health care services who expects good care as a return for his or her investment. Similar to other industries, health care organizations are forced to compete for consumer dollars, and if they are to succeed, they need to convince consumers that they can provide valuable services to improve their health status. The definition of good care is evolving from a subjective opinion to the objectivity of using Centers for Medicare and Medicaid Services (CMS) comparative data that analyzes outcomes by disease as a yardstick for value.

Information about the value of care at hospitals comes to the public through report cards of explicitly defined quality indicators that identify the best performers. Performance is explained to the consumer through such indicators as mortality rates, measurements on disease management that describe best practices, and increased competency that is related to a surgeon's experience (that is, volume) for a particular procedure. Consumers have also been introduced to concepts of unexpected mortality in a hospital and issues related to patient safety, such as hospital-acquired infections. This information provides value to the patient and economic incentives to hospitals to eliminate or reduce unsafe practices.

Hospitals are required to collect and submit data about these clinical and safety indicators so that information can be made available to the public. Until recently, hospital administrators did not recognize the value of transparency; many still believe that public reporting hurts hospital reputations and does not improve care. Administrators who resist the push toward transparency believe that data collection efforts and public reporting initiatives simply increase expenses. Quality is seen as a remote value that their organization should have—but only when money becomes available to the hospital. Quality is thought to be external to the operation of the hospital and has little to do with improving cash flow. Value-based purchasing, attempts by those who spend money on health care services to monitor, measure, and improve the quality of care they receive for their expenditure is often not accepted as relevant to health care.

Through data collection initiatives, however, the federal government is hoping to focus increased attention on implementing safety processes. By financially rewarding those organizations who comply with the indicators, the government is trying to change the culture of health care, to incorporate evidence-based medicine, and to standardize the treatment of specific patient populations. Both the public awareness of safety measures and the government focus on data encourage physicians to adopt new practices, to consider evidence from large databases, and to respond to aggregated data from within their own organizations.

Health care organizations are being forced to change the way they do business, and the way they think about the value of the services they provide because the economic structure of reimbursement is undergoing change. Hospitals are expected to provide indicators that quality care is delivered, quality care as defined by specific government-endorsed indicators. Services that are required to repair poor care on selected conditions might not be reimbursed. Poor care costs the hospitals money. Quality care provides value.

Because health care expenditure is reaching critical proportions, and because health care services have been exposed as potentially dangerous, problem ridden, and ineffective, the government and other organizations are stepping in to attempt to improve care and control costs. Improving the management of chronic diseases makes economic as well as clinical sense. Understanding disease management from a population point of view makes better sense than treating specific individuals idiosyncratically. As governments and health care organizations search for ways to better manage expenses, a definition of value is emerging. Value is inextricably linked to good care. Good care is defined through quality measures. Quality measures are objective and explicit indicators of care. Large government initiatives, such as pay for performance and never events, connect good outcomes with financial rewards.

Therefore the provision of good care is based on measures derived from evidence-based medicine. Performance is defined through quality indicators of disease. Value, as defined by Centers for Medicare and Medicaid Services (CMS), means getting good results for patients. Good results lead to increased financial rewards. By requiring hospitals to better manage chronic diseases and to reward measures that go beyond the acute stage of treatment, the CMS and other organizations are stressing the value of good care. There is little return on investment when patients are readmitted due to poor treatment, inadequate discharge instructions, or ineffective education and flawed communication. By focusing on the entire continuum of care, from the emergency department visit through hospital discharge to home care, clinicians and administrators are required to address questions about the quality of care that they have never asked before.

Senior leadership, the C suite, has begun to take an interest in the measurements of the quality of care that lead to communication with the clinical staff and focus on documentation and obstacles for proper documentation. However, leaders are not yet focused on the processes that prevent their organizations from reaching the top decile on quality indicators. Programs such as pay for performance, which link compliance with quality indicators and financial rewards, are redefining value for administrators. Compliance with required measures depends on accurate documentation that specific variables have been incorporated into the treatment plan. Documentation is based on accurate data collection and processes for reporting data. Therefore, administrative leadership is beginning to recognize the value of quality methodologies to support data collection and analysis and compliance for improved performance. Because good care and good outcomes are rewarded, administrators and clinicians are beginning to recognize the link between compliance with prescribed quality indicators and improved care. These changes are adding value to health care.

Value is measured by matching expectation to results. Today's chief executive officers (CEOs) and chief financial officers (CFOs) are incorporating concepts from pay for performance and never events initiatives into the budget. They are asking questions about lack of compliance with timely aspirin administration, barriers to lowering infection rates, and appropriateness of patient admission. Databases have been developed to help answer these questions. These kinds of questions, once the purview only of the clinician, are helping to integrate the various groups involved in the delivery of care. Relationships need to be formed among administrative and clinical staff, between clinician and environmental staff, between the community and the hospital. Integrating these once distinct domains increases value as defined as increased quality and improved finances.

As traditional barriers begin to break down between those who make financial decisions and those who deliver clinical care, communication is improving. The discussion of quality variables has promoted a common language. Now administrators, clinicians, government agencies, and patients all inquire about infection rates, mortality rates, specifics of disease management such as aspirin administration. We are all talking about the same thing: improving patient safety, documenting quality care, and increasing organizational efficiency. Documentation of care as the basis for reimbursement is now supported by administration. There is value to keeping an accurate medical record; there is value to transferring information across the continuum of care; and there is value associated with reducing adverse events and sentinel events. Everyone involved in the health care organization is expected to participate in these discussions. With increased transparency, data reveal the details of care processes; those details are everyone's business. CEOs can no longer remain aloof from clinical care.

As the focus of reimbursement becomes increasingly directed toward value-based purchasing, quality will shift from an abstract concept to a concept integral to the process of care. The government is educating the public about the appropriate management of disease; government programs are attempting to redirect administration and leadership about the value of compliance with evidence-based measures through a reward system and the concept of not paying for care that leads to poor outcomes that should have been prevented. Hospital leaders are pressuring clinicians to participate in the documentation efforts, data collection methods, and improved communication initiatives because such compliance is rewarded. With health care organizations competing for market share, hospitals with poor publicity, negative media reports because of poor outcomes, low or no reimbursement for never events will suffer financially. Value resides in good care. However, for hospitals, the shift takes time and reculturation.

Today the boards of trustees of health care organizations receive two separate reports, one on quality and one on finance. Education about the relationship between the two separate domains needs to be established. The CMS, insurers, business, and industry organizations are introducing quality as intrinsic to financial success. Medical schools need to focus their training on the relationship among process, outcomes, and defects. Poor performance will be defined as an expense that hospital administrators won't tolerate. Good to excellent performance will be defined as a measure of financial success. Clinicians have to become part of the administrative team; they can no longer stand apart wrapped in specialized knowledge. The pay-for-performance and never events initiative go beyond mere compliance with measures by the individual physician. The concepts should be used as a framework to improve upon the care as system and process issues.

When there are errors, mistakes, and undesired events, the private domain of the mortality and morbidity (M&M) conference is no longer a viable method to address clinical issues. Errors require time and commitment from many members of the health care organization to devise better processes and avoid future errors. Again, documentation is central, serving as the basis for the review of care and the analysis of flaws and gaps. The medical record is a database describing the care and the relationship among all the disciplines who are involved in the patient's care. The electronic medical record will increase access to information in that key information will be transformed into data; that data can be used for analysis, to assess and measure care, and to improve.

Administrative data collection efforts such as cardiac mortality or transplant registers have created large databases for analysis. Now specifics of diagnosis, mortality, and some complications can be compared across the nation, with risk-adjusted benchmarks providing information about how one organization compares to another. These benchmarks define the best, according to private groups such as HealthGrades, that become the window for the public to look into the hospital's medical care.

The gold standard of care is being established, and it is evolving as measurements on process of disease, care, and outcome become available. The measurements will be correlated with financial measures. Such concepts as waste, overuse, underuse, and appropriate use need to be redefined. Organizations that fall below the desired level will generate poor publicity and will need to explain and justify poor performance. Thus government efforts to educate the public and force documentation of quality measures are driving new economic forces that will lead to new measures of care. When leadership receives reports that their organization falls short, they inquire why. That inquiry leads to analysis of processes, identification of gaps and risks, and improvement efforts. That inquiry leads to increased value as long as the process of care is improved.

Measures are central to analyzing gaps in care via benchmarks and control charts. CMS has targeted the chronic diseases, such as heart failure, and supplied specific variables for managing care. The focus is not only on processes but also on results, such as readmission rates. Readmission may be an indication of poor discharge planning. As understanding of care is enhanced, expectations for improved outcomes are higher. High expectations by the public will focus administration on improving care processes.

Value is related to improvement in care, reduced inefficiencies, and enhanced income for hospitals. Finance and quality are inexorably intertwined. Financial success is dependent on good care and good management of the processes that govern the clinical team. Those involved in health care should applaud and support such efforts and incorporate quality management processes for superior performance. Everyone will benefit.

REFERENCES

Agency for Health Care Policy and Research. *Clinical Practice Guidelines No. 3.* Rockville, MD: U.S. Department of Health and Human Services, 1994.

Aguayo, R. *Dr. Deming: The American Who Taught the Japanese About Quality.* New York: Simon & Schuster, 1990.

Annandale, E., Elston, M. A., and Prior, L. *Medical Work, Medical Knowledge and Health Care.* Malden, MA: Blackwell, 2004.

Berwick, D. M. "Continuous Improvement as an Ideal in Health Care." In N. O. Graham (ed.), *Quality in Health Care: Theory, Application, and Evolution.* Gaithersburg, MD: Aspen, 1995.

Champy, J. *X-Engineering for the Corporation: Reinventing Your Business in the Digital Age.* New York: Warner Books, 2002.

Chowdhury, S. *The Power of Six Sigma.* Chicago: Dearborn, 2001.

Cockerham, W. C. *Medical Sociology.* Upper Saddle River, NJ: Prentice Hall, 1989.

Codman, E. A. *A Study in Hospital Efficiency as Demonstrated by the Case Report of the First Five Years of a Private Hospital.* Oakbrook Terrace, IL: Joint Commission on Accreditation of Healthcare Organizations, 1996.

Colen, B. D. *O.R.: The True Story of 24 Hours in a Hospital Operating Room.* New York: Dutton, 1993.

Dlugacz, Y. D. Foreword, *Getting the Board on Board: What Your Board Needs to Know About Quality and Patient Safety.* Oakbrook Terrace, IL: Joint Commission Resources, 2007.

Dlugacz, Y. D. "Handling a Surprise JCAHO Inspection." *Modern Healthcare,* November 14, 2005. S10–S12.

Dlugacz, Y. D. "High-Quality Care Reaps Financial Rewards." *HFMA (Healthcare Financial Management Association) Strategic Financial Planning,* Summer 2007. 8–9.

Dlugacz, Y. D. "Keep It Clean!" *Health Care Link,* August 23, 2005, S10–S11.

Dlugacz, Y. D. *Measuring Health Care: Using Quality Data for Operational, Financial and Clinical Improvement.* San Francisco: Jossey-Bass, 2006.

Dlugacz, Y. D. "Patient Safety and Quality, Role of Governance." *Asian Hospital & Healthcare Management,* 2007, *14,* 10–12.

Dlugacz, Y. D. Review of "Methods of Family Research: Biographies of Research Projects, Vol. II." *Readings: Journal of Reviews and Commentary in Mental Health,* May 1990.

Dlugacz, Y. D., Restifo, A., and Greenwood, A. *The Quality Handbook for Health Care Organizations: A Manager's Guide to Tools and Programs.* San Francisco: Jossey-Bass, 2004.

Dlugacz, Y. D., Restifo, A., and Nelson, K. "Implementing Evidence-Based Guidelines and Reporting Results Through a Quality Metric." *Patient Safety and Quality Healthcare,* 2005, *2*(2), 40–42.

Dlugacz, Y. D., Rosati, R. J., and Tortolani, A. J. "Communicating Quality Assurance Data to Trustees." *Quality Times* (Hospital Association of New York State), March 1991, 9–11.

Dlugacz, Y. D., and Stier, L. "More Quality Bang for Your Healthcare Buck." *Journal of Nursing Care Quality,* 2005, *20*(2), 174–181.

Dlugacz, Y. D., Stier, L., and Greenwood, A. "Changing the System: A Quality Management Approach to Pressure Injuries." *Journal of Healthcare Quality,* 2001, *23*(5), 15–20.

Dlugacz, Y. D., and Sweetapple, C., "An Innovative Approach to a Care Pathway for Total Hip Replacement." *Asian Hospital & Healthcare Management*, 2008, *17*, 14–17.

Dlugacz, Y. D., and others. "Expanding a Performance Improvement Initiative in Critical Care." *Joint Commission Journal on Quality Improvement*, 2002, *28*, 419–434.

Dlugacz, Y. D., and others. "Safety Strategies to Prevent Suicide in Multiple Health Care Environments." *Joint Commission Journal on Quality and Safety*, 2003, *29*(6), 267–277.

Dlugacz, Y. D., and others. *Understanding Publicly Reported Quality Measures.* New York: HANYS Quality Institute, December 2007.

Donabedian, A. "The Role of Outcomes in Quality Assessment and Assurance." In N. O. Graham (ed.), *Quality in Health Care: Theory, Application, and Evolution.* Gaithersburg, MD: Aspen, 1995, 198–209.

Gawande, A. *Complications: A Surgeon's Notes on an Imperfect Science.* New York: Metropolitan Books, 2002.

George, M. L. *Lean Six Sigma for Service.* New York: McGraw-Hill, 2003.

Halm, E. A., and others. "Limited Impact of a Multicenter Intervention to Improve the Quality and Efficiency of Pneumonia Care." *Chest*, 2004, *126*, 100–107.

Hussain, E., and Kao, E. "Medication Safety and Transfusion Errors in the ICU and Beyond." *Critical Care Clinics*, 2005, *21*(1), 91–110.

Joint Commission on Accreditation of Healthcare Organizations. *Failure Mode and Effects Analysis in Health Care: Proactive Risk Reduction.* Joint Commission Resources. Oakbrook Terrace, IL: Joint Commission on Accreditation of Healthcare Organizations, 2002.

Joint Commission on Accreditation of Healthcare Organizations. *Florence Nightingale: Measuring Hospital Outcomes.* Joint Commission Resources. Oakbrook Terrace, IL: Joint Commission on Accreditation of Healthcare Organizations, 1999.

Joint Commission on Accreditation of Healthcare Organizations. *Framework for Improving Performance: From Principles to Practice.* Joint Commission Resources. Oakbrook Terrace, IL: Joint Commission on Accreditation of Healthcare Organizations, 1994.

Joint Commission on Accreditation of Healthcare Organizations. *From Practice to Paper: Documentation for Hospitals.* Joint Commission Resources. Oakbrook Terrace, IL: Joint Commission on Accreditation of Healthcare Organizations, 2002.

Joint Commission on Accreditation of Healthcare Organizations. *Hospital Accreditation Standards.* Joint Commission Resources. Oakbrook Terrace, IL: Joint Commission on Accreditation of Healthcare Organizations, 2002.

Juran, J. M. *Juran on Quality by Design: The New Steps for Planning Quality into Goods and Services.* New York: Free Press, 1992.

Kohn, L. T., Corrigan, J. M., and Donaldson, M. S. (eds.). *To Err Is Human: Building a Safer Health System.* Washington, DC: National Academies Press, 1999.

Kumar, Sanjaya. *Fatal Care: Survive in the U.S. Health System.* Minneapolis: Igi Press, 2008.

Lustbader, D., Cooper, D., Reiser, P., Dlugacz, Y. D., and Fein, A. "Methodology for Improved ICU Resource Utilization and Quality of Care." *Chest*, 1998, *114*(4), 254S.

Lustbader, D., Dlugacz, Y. D., Weissman, G., Stier, L., and Fein, A. "Regional Benchmarking for Critical Care: Methodology for Quality Improvement." *Chest*, 1998, *114*(4), 342S.

Lustbader, D., Sparrow, P., Silver, A., Dlugacz, Y. D., and Fein, A. "Ventilator Care in a Large Hospital Network." *Chest*, 1998, *114*(4), 343.

McKinlay, J. B., Lin, T., Freund, K., and Moskowitz, M. "The Unexpected Influence of Physician Attributes on Clinical Decisions: Results of an Experiment." *Journal of Health and Social Behavior*, 2002, *43*(1), 92–106.

Milstein, A., and others. "Improving the Safety of Health Care: The Leapfrog Initiative. The Leapfrog Group." *Effective Clinical Practice*, 2000, *5*, 313–316.

The New England Journal of Medicine. *Quality of Care: Selections from the New England Journal of Medicine.* Waltham, MA: Massachusetts Medical Society, 1997.

Parsons, T. *The Social System.* New York: Free Press, 1951.

Report to the Congress: Promoting Greater Efficiency in Medicare, June 2007.

Robertson, S., Lesser, M. L., Kohn, N., Cooper, D. J., and Dlugacz, Y. D. "Statistical and Methodological Issues in the Evaluation of Case Management Studies." *Journal of Health Care Quality,* 1996, *18*(6), 25–31.

Rosati, R., and Dlugacz, Y. D. "The Use of Data Analysis and Feedback to Manage the Length of Stay of Medically Treated Neurology Patients." Philadelphia: Society for Medical Decision Making, 1991.

Spath, P. L. "Reducing Errors Through Work System Improvements." In P. L. Spath (ed.), *Error Reduction in Health Care: A Systems Approach to Improving Patient Safety.* San Francisco: Jossey-Bass, 2000.

Stier, L., and others. "Reinforcing Organization-Wide Pressure Ulcer Reduction on High-Risk Geriatric Inpatient Units." *Outcomes Management,* 2004, *8*(1), 28–32.

Studer, Q. *Hardwiring Excellence: Purpose, Worthwhile Work, and Making a Difference.* Gulf Breeze, FL: Fire Starter, 2003.

Timmermans, S., and Angell, A. "Evidence-Based Medicine, Clinical Uncertainty, and Learning to Doctor." *Journal of Health and Social Behavior,* 2001, *42*(4), 342–359.

Weinstock, M. S., and Dlugacz, Y. D. "Integration of Emergency Department Care with the Hospital Process." *Quality Assurance in Emergency Medicine* (2nd ed.) Irving, TX: American College of Emergency Physicians.

White, K. *An Introduction to the Sociology of Health and Illness.* Thousand Oaks, CA: Sage, 2002.

Williams, S. C., Schmaltz, S. P., Morton, D. J., Koss, R. G., and Loeb, J. M. "Quality of Care in U.S. Hospitals as Reflected by Standardized Measures, 2002–2004." *New England Journal of Medicine,* 2005, *353,* 255–264.

Zussman, R. *Intensive Care: Medical Ethics and the Medical Profession.* Chicago: University of Chicago Press, 1992.

USEFUL WEB SITES

CENTERS FOR MEDICARE AND MEDICAID SERVICES

www.cms.hhs.gov
The Web site of the Centers for Medicare and Medicaid Services (CMS) provides links to information about the "never events" and other quality-of-care patient safety initiatives. CMS is the federal agency that is part of the Department of Health and Human Services (HHS) and administers Medicare, Medicaid, SCHIP (State Children's Health Insurance), and several other health-related programs.

CMS HOSPITAL COMPARE

www.hospitalcompare.hhs.gov
Quality measures are publicly reported on the CMS Hospital Compare Web site, which compares hospitals according to safety rankings.

CMS VALUE-DRIVEN HEALTH CARE

www.hhs.gov/valuedriven
CMS's efforts to encourage improvement in all aspects of quality, including patient safety, and increase the efficiency of health care services, has led to its value-based purchasing (VBP) initiative, which incorporates performance-based financial incentives and public reporting of quality information. This site also provides information about the movement toward transparency.

COMMITTEE TO REDUCE INFECTION DEATHS

www.hospitalinfection.org
A nonprofit educational group, the Committee to Reduce Infection Deaths (RID), collects and publishes information about hospital-acquired infections that result in death. RID educates the public about steps they can take to reduce the risk of acquiring a hospital infection.

INSTITUTE FOR HEALTHCARE IMPROVEMENT

www.ihi.org

The Web site of the Institute for Healthcare Improvement (IHI) offers information on various initiatives, including the 5 million lives campaign. The IHI is an independent not-for-profit organization that promotes patient safety programs around the world.

JOINT COMMISSION

www.jointcommission.org

The Joint Commission Web site provides information about sentinel events, patient safety initiatives, such as the national patient safety goals, and various performance measurement initiatives, as well as the standards for hospital accreditation.

LEAPFROG GROUP

www.leapfroggroup.org

The Leapfrog Group provides information to the public about health care quality and hospital safety, ranked according to procedure, in order to encourage comparison. In addition, the Web site explains its criteria for ranking and how it is attempting to influence hospitals to improve their delivery of care through financial incentives.

INDEX

Page references followed by *fig* indicate illustrated figure.